D0431605

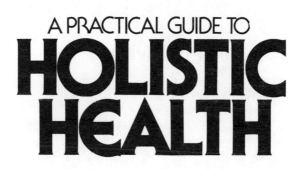

A PRACTICAL GUIDE TO
HOLISTIC HEALTH

A PRACTICAL GUIDE TO
HOLISTIC HEALTH

BY SWAMI RAMA

Revised Edition

The Himalayan International Institute
Honesdale, Pennsylvania

Library of Congress Catalog Card Number: 80-81598

ISBN: 0-89389-066-9
ISBN: 0-89389-065-0 pbk

© 1980 by
The Himalayan International Institute of Yoga Science and Philosophy
of the U.S.A.

Second Edition 1980
Second printing 1983

THE HIMALAYAN INTERNATIONAL INSTITUTE OF YOGA
SCIENCE AND PHILOSOPHY
RD 1, Box 88
Honesdale, Pennsylvania 18431

Printed in the United States of America.

All suffering that afflicts the mind or the body has ignorance for its cause, and all happiness has its basis in clear, scientific knowledge. *Charaka*

Contents

Introduction

As a nation we are approaching a crisis in health care. In a country blessed with abundant material wealth, we continue to be burdened with a plague of chronic disease. Medical expenses have become overwhelming, and there seems to be no promise of their slowing. The problem seems baffling, its solution unsolvable. Yet we must begin to face up to the facts.

Half of us will die from "hardening of the arteries," and another twenty five per cent will end our lives with cancer. Millions more are suffering right now with arthritis, respiratory disease and alcoholism. Disregarding infant mortality, our life expectancies have changed little since 1900, though medical expenses have increased by over thirty times since that date. Technological advances have increased dramatically in the last decade, and each passing year brings a revolutionary surgical procedure or a new wonder drug. Yet despite all of these discoveries the attainment of physical health eludes our grasp.

In the realm of our mental well-being, the situation seems no brighter. Many of us feel emotionally unbalanced, depressed, and dissatisfied with our lot. We have one of the highest rates of suicide, mental illness, and other serious social problems. Nearly one million persons are now being treated in a variety of mental facilities, and many more are incarcerated in prisons, detention homes, and reform schools.

We blame the deteriorating state of our health and the society as a whole on external factors. We say that we live in a very stressful world, and stress is pointed to as the cause of many of our illnesses. We say that with all the economic uncertainties, high-pressured competitiveness and social complexities, it is impossible to alleviate or improve our present condition. Because we don't take the time to eat right, exercise, and do those things that are best for us, we rationalize that when sickness comes, the doctor is always there to help make us better. This way of thinking has led to the indiscriminate consumption of medicines promising quick and instant relief: last year over thirty-eight million pounds of aspirin were consumed, and over five hundred million dollars were spent on one type of tranquilizer alone.

Clearly, this way of living has proven far from satisfactory. We have learned to ignore the cues that our bodies and minds were trying to tell us about our health. By the time many of us become aware of our problems it is already too late to do anything about them.

Many express the opinions: "So what? What's the big deal? After all, what else can we do? We have the best hospitals, the smartest doctors, and the most advanced drugs at our disposal, so what else can be done?" Indeed, this may be true. However, there exist societies today that have no doctors, hospitals, or sophisticated technological hardware, in which the lifespan of many of their citizens goes beyond one hundred years. Senility is rare, and most demonstrate heightened wisdom in their later years. In these societies there are no psychologists, social workers, or policemen either. Mental illness, divorce, suicide, and crime are virtually non-existent.

The question then presents itself: if it is possible for some to live long and healthy lives, then why are we with all of our material advantages having so many problems? More importantly, what can we do to make our lives healthier and our enjoyment of life more fulfilling?

In all of our activities we are looking for happiness, but we apparently lack the knowledge to attain this goal. Rather than blame society for our problems—a difficult institution to alter—we must begin to look at ourselves. What can we do as individuals to attain this state of well-being?

It is to this specific issue that Swami Rama addresses himself in this book. As a scholar of Eastern and Western medicine, psychology, and philosophy, he is eminently qualified to attempt such a project. Compiled from a series of lectures, this book simply and eloquently shares his knowledge and expertise. By integrating Western science with the traditional wisdom of the sages, Swami Rama presents a systematic self-training program; application of these principles will lead us to the state of wellness and happiness which he calls holistic health.

Holistic health is shown to mean more than physical or mental fitness; it is a state where one understands the purpose of life. In order to reach this goal it is necessary to follow certain laws that have been validated throughout the ages, having found expression in the writings of all the great spiritual traditions. As one begins to delve into the idea of holistic health he begins to see these words as a paradigm for a much broader concept. The goal of each of us is to realize who we are and why we are here; to reach these answers we must go on a journey of exploration and seeking. Traveling this route may be difficult, and like the pilgrim beginning his ten-thousand-mile-trek, we must begin one step at a time. Yet we are fortunate—the map has been provided by those who have walked this way before us.

It is the hope of all of us to attain this state of holistic health. As Swami Rama so masterfully exemplifies, the power to do so lies within each of us. It is merely a matter of cultivating our determination and will. By taking proper care of our bodies, regulating our breath, and learning to control our emotions, each of us can rediscover our inner source of physical well-being, emotional contentment, and everlasting peace. The path has been illuminated—it is now our responsibility to take the first step.

Matthew Monsein, M.D.
May 16, 1978

1

What is
Holistic Health?

Our modern civilization claims to be very productive, creative and resourceful, but a hundred years ago we did not have many of the diseases that exist today. Every day more diseases are being created. For although we are alive, the majority of us experience only the art of existing. Very few of us have really cultivated that technique which is called the art of living. The reason for this is that life today has become very artificial. Man never stops to consider that he may have gone too far by ignoring his natural resources and by depending on artificial means. Living by artificial means gradually decreases natural resistances and this obsession makes modern man suffer more and more. Man's whole life seems to be kept busy in trying to get rid of self-created suffering. Is there nothing higher for human beings to obtain than freedom from these ailments?

There is no remedy in any system of medicine for such a self-created condition except to be aware of the fact that it is the individual who creates these miseries for himself and that only he can learn how to prevent them. With the bounty of nature outside and the center of consciousness within, one should be living in health and harmony, but having built boundaries, both externally and internally, the direct contact with these forces has been lost. All human beings have the inner potential and skill to be completely healthy, but in today's world, because of the social and economic pressures, human beings have forgotten that all things happen deep within before they appear on the physical and mental levels. One must understand his inner skills and resources and use them as much as possible in order to insure perfect health.

By first paying attention to the physical being, one becomes aware that all his actions, emotions, and feelings are governed from within by the conscious and unconscious minds. Finally, one realizes that his mental aspect of health is more important than the physical, and that the spiritual aspect of health is of greater importance than either of these. When one starts paying attention to the various zones of his being and learns to transcend them, the most subtle level of existence comes into consciousness. Ultimately, one becomes aware of the center of consciousness within, that which flows outward in various degrees and grades. This particular level is called spiritual health. Those who understand this are practicing the art of living and being. One who remains constantly aware of this center enjoys all the gifts of life.

The ancients were aware of the fact that human beings suffer on various levels: physical, mental, and spiritual. They did much research, and if modern man would learn how to modify and apply that research, he would not be as unhealthy and insecure as he is today. The Upanishads say that if one possesses both *avidya* (mundane, temporal knowledge) and *vidya* (spiritual knowledge), he can remain happy, successfully cross the mire of delusion, and be liberated. The ancients emphasized the necessity of holistic health which means to understand the entire human being. This study is as ancient as human life. Only a few texts survive which describe the practical steps for achieving physical, mental, and spiritual health, and these are understood by only a small number of accomplished yogis and scholars. I was taught some of these manuscripts, and I want to pass on this knowledge.

In studying health, one learns biological, physiological, psychological, and philosophical concepts, but I want to explain an entirely different concept. I want to discuss holistic health, which includes all of the above, as seen from the yoga viewpoint. I will describe the health practices which have been taught in the Himalayas for centuries and give a few simple and subtle points which will help in attaining a good and healthy life. In doing this I will examine health on the physical, mental, and spiritual levels. The yoga approach to health is extremely simple, logical, and practical. It lays stress on the words *Yuktahar viharasya*—eating and living as they should be done. By simply studying one's own capacity and learning how to regulate one's dietary habits, external activities, and thinking process, it is possible for one to gain control over his life and remain healthy. This does not mean that one must do anything unnatural or impossible; there need not be restrictions, but given the information in these lessons, one can decide what is best for himself, and implement whatever changes he chooses, practicing them according to his own capacity.

The yoga practices described in the ancient manuscripts are not just physical; they are mental and spiritual too, for yoga is the science of self-effort, of self-examination, and of self-awareness. It is a scientific discipline perfected over millennia. The yoga techniques work. They have been proven and validated by many. By sincerely and honestly following these simple rules, one will achieve success. As one practices, he will begin to see and feel how much he has accomplished through his own daily efforts. In this way, he will understand the way to attainment.

The ancient manuals to which I am referring explain the science of living and discuss the techniques for extending the life span by means of a system called Ayurvedic medicine. *Ayur* means "age," and *veda* means "science of." Ayurvedic medicine originated to control the aging process. I have heard people say that they are very intelligent, but what happens to their intelligence after they reach the age of seventy? In our society today people who are over seventy or eighty years old are put into a nursing home. The theory is that they do not communicate well and since they can no longer care for themselves, they are useless and a burden. Modern man loses his intelligence before he gets old, but old people should actually be the wisest and most capable of teaching since they have experienced more. In ancient times men did not lose intelligence as they grew old. On the contrary, the more they aged, the wiser they became.

This is the difference: we grow old and lose our intelligence; they grew with age and were called wise. They understood more because they knew of the power of living. We have lost this knowledge.

Many modern academicians say people were ignorant in ancient times, but I don't agree with them. The ancients knew much about life. What is more, their science was very sophisticated. Surgical operations, for instance, were being performed successfully by Indian physicians hundreds of years ago, and the Chinese knew about the principles of vaccination centuries before Jenner's "revolutionary" discovery. Yet despite these skills, the ancients did not disregard the importance of prevention. The major emphasis of the ancient texts is on a holistic approach. Diet and proper elimination were stressed. Correct breathing and self-control were taught, and the influence of climate was carefully considered. Their therapies were tailored to fit the requirements and the constitution of the individual. Because ancient medicine emphasized prevention rather than "druggation," modern science is only now beginning to verify their findings.

Unfortunately, most modern researchers still believe in replacement, not in prevention. They would rather spend billions of dollars looking for the cure for cancer, or a way to successfully replace a diseased heart with that of a monkey, than understand the laws of health and wellness. They do not realize that preventive medicine is the best, the easiest, and the most rewarding approach. Getting sick and then getting rid of sickness is a painful experience as well as a waste of time and energy. One should learn to look after the body so that it does not become a source of constant pain and misery. One should cultivate and practice those skills which insure health, rather than fall victim to those which perpetuate disease. There are two ways of doing this—one is external and the other is internal. Most of us look after our health by depending on the external sources, but physical health means much more than merely developing huge muscles, or eating the proper diet, or even taking super-fortified vitamins and mineral supplements. For if a human being learns to develop only his muscles and does not realize his mental capacities, then for lack of this mental willpower and inner strength, he suffers and always remains cowardly and insecure. Pain, fear, and suffering will continue to exist, so it is important for one to be aware of the internal environment and not to be solely dependent on the external one, for it is inner contentment and mental satisfaction which are the real keys to health.

The time has come for man to realize that he is not a body alone. He is a breathing being and a thinking being too—a unique individual made up of complex emotions, appetites, and desires. So even if one spent years studying nutrition, physiology, or even going through medical school, the knowledge he would gain would be neither completely satisfying nor completely useful in helping to maintain perfect health. This is because that which is related to the body, that which is material, is not all there is. The body is merely a covering outside the mind, and the mind is a covering outside the center of consciousness within. It is very important to be aware that the body is a tool and not the entire self. Although the body is the most gross tool, it is the instrument used in day-to-day life, and through it one learns many things. So it is still very important and necessary and must be properly taken care of.

With the body's help man can fly to the moon, but he cannot fathom the deepest levels of his own consciousness. As long as his consciousness remains arrested in body awareness, man will not achieve any other level of consciousness. As long as he identifies with his body only, it will create many problems and obstacles for him. It is only after the body is transformed to a useful tool that it can be used as a means for right expression and for communicating with others. Often when the body is sick, one begins to pay so much attention to it that he cannot communicate with others as he should. For when the body experiences pain, all one can do is focus on the pain. Instead of gaining knowledge, one has pain. He cannot share the pain with anyone else, not even those with whom he shares his joy. No matter how much others love him, they cannot share his pain. They can only console him by diverting his mind.

Life means relationships, and without communication, relationships and life both will crumble. Without a healthy mind, it is not possible for a good body to become a good tool for communication. Even modern athletes are becoming aware that without a sound mind it is difficult to have a good body. Interaction with others needs a healthy body and a sound mind. An unhealthy body keeps the mental faculties busy on the physical level only, and one cannot think of anything else but his body. Pain implies selfishness. It is impossible to care about another when one is continuously in pain. Every human being has something to offer to others, and if a human being is not capable of offering his services to others because of pain, then he is unhealthy. To eliminate the pain he must find another dimension of life higher than the body.

When a human being starts to analyze himself, starts to understand himself, he knows that he is not the body alone. He has lived with the body so much and has been told so often that his body is who he is, that he constantly identifies with it. This belief is so strong that no matter how much you read or study, no matter how much someone teaches you differently, your entire consciousness comes back to the body alone.

Actually, the body is nothing more than an airport where the plane called the inner being lands. Stop reading for a moment. Try to get out of your chair. Watch carefully. You will soon realize that it is not your body which does the standing, but it is something else within that orders the mass of flesh and bones to stand. The body is merely an instrument which obeys orders. When one examines himself carefully, he finds that there is a center within that has the power to make him stand firmly, to sit quietly, to move or wait if he wants. This center has the potential to be one's greatest ally or one's worst enemy; it is the source of health or dis-ease.

Attitude is the most important factor in realizing health. Many people actually want to be unhealthy, sad, and miserable. They develop that tendency more and more until they create that personality for themselves. Later on they become helpless and do not want to accept the fact that they themselves are responsible for their ill health. It is important for people to become aware of the fact that staying healthy is not merely a matter of good diet, taking vitamins, or even doing proper physical exercise. More crucial than any of these factors is keeping a healthy state of mind.

Good mental health cannot be disturbed no matter what happens. Many people today say that they spend so much time eating, sleeping, talking to others, and carrying out other duties that it is not possible for them to attain the goal of human life in this lifetime. So they want to know about previous lives in order to understand their link with the past. It is a natural tendency of human beings to brood on past experiences. It is also their nature to imagine what the future might hold for them. But when they spend so much time thinking about the past or worrying about the future, they never learn how to be here and now. They cannot understand it; they cannot realize it, and no one can teach them how to be here and now. The moment they think of now, it is no longer there. One cannot think of now and live in the now at the same time, but once one understands what "now" means, he comes out of the past and future and learns to live in the present. Those who learn to live in the moment and have a purpose do not know what sadness is, nor do they sway with the moods or phases of life.

There are three categories of people traveling through

the procession of life: time oriented, goal oriented, and purpose oriented. Time oriented people move in the world without understanding why they are moving. They do not have any true vision of the future. They spend their lives fantasizing some idyllic future or analyzing triumphs or defeats from the past. They lack a sense of discipline and purpose. Because they are continually living in their projections of the way things might have been, or could be, they fail to appreciate things the way they are, and are thus forever dissatisfied. For such people, staying healthy and finding success is difficult.

The second category of people is those who are goal oriented. They can physically and mentally discipline themselves to a certain extent, and they can conduct their duties according to circumstances, but their vision remains limited. Their goals are confined to worldly attainments such as, "I will have a house, a wife, a car, a job, and many other comforts." For lack of a higher purpose their lives remain oriented toward material goals. They think that these things will satisfy them and fulfill the purpose of life, but after attaining them, they feel lost because they do not know why they had sought them in the first place.

The third category of people is comprised of those few individuals who are purpose oriented. Whatever they think, speak, and do is in accordance with their purpose in life. They regulate their habits and know that physical and mental health are not two different things, but are inseparable units which are essential for maintaining holistic health. For them maintaining good physical and mental health is like preserving two fine instruments which can be used to carry out the purpose of life. What label one attaches to this purpose—happiness, perfection, health, a state of tranquility, *nirvana, samadhi*, Godhead—is immaterial. The people of this last category are rare, but they are healthy in all respects.

Thus it is clear that the basis of holistic health lies in one's understanding the purpose of his life and learning how to achieve that purpose. There are many questions human beings want to answer. However, it is only when they are sick or they don't have all the normal amenities of life, or when they are befallen by a personal tragedy that they begin asking, "Why am I here? What is the purpose of my life? From where have I come? Where will I go?" These are not cultural questions. They are not social or economic questions either. These are inborn questions common to every human being and they arise when one starts examining life. Everyone has to face these questions sooner or later. Without answers to these questions, mere physical health or mental soundness will not fulfill the purpose of life. An emptiness, a void, and a feeling of dissatisfaction within will still remain. For instance, after attempting many experiments along the path of happiness, couples frequently do not know why they are still unhappy. Although they live together, love each other, are sincere and honest, and do their duties, they are not fully satisfied. They do not know why they are unhappy because they still do not know the purpose of their lives. It is very important to realize the source of their unhappiness so that their unconscious minds do not create problems and keep them from being free. For if one knows where he has come from and why he has come, and if he has no fear of death, then he will enjoy life, even on the sensory level. Commonly people cannot really enjoy their pleasures because they are more concerned with their fears. They worry: "What will happen if this thing is snatched from me? What will happen if one of us dies? What will happen if something suddenly occurs?" Fear is our greatest enemy, and if allowed to develop excessively, it even threatens our sense of self-preservation. To succumb to fear is like committing suicide. But with human beings there is always fear, always something that does not allow us to fully enjoy life's privileges. Only when one can attain a state which is free from fear can he enjoy all things within and without.

I am not talking about emotional or ignorant fearlessness. For instance, I once saw a bull rush in anger to attack an oncoming train. He killed himself, of course. I am talking about that fearlessness which can be attained by understanding life as much as possible through mental concepts and behavior. Human beings are perfectly equipped with all the necessary resources to attain this state of fearlessness, and happiness, wisdom, and enlightenment can only be achieved from that state. Otherwise, happiness is only a word that one knows how to spell, while he cannot understand what it really is until he attains freedom from all anxieties.

To achieve this understanding one must have a practical philosophy of life. This begins to evolve the moment one realizes that it has been missing. Buddha developed a very practical approach to life. He said there are four noble truths. If one becomes aware of them he will be able to understand the whole philosophy of human life. Buddha says first that one has to accept that there is misery in life. Don't ignore it; instead analyze and understand it. Second, he says that misery has a cause. Third, he says that there is a way of eliminating the cause. And fourth, he claims, there is a state which is free from all miseries, but as long as the human mind is going through pain and misery, it can never realize the truth. So Buddha says that if one learns to face life's miseries and become a witness rather than a victim, then he will begin to enjoy life. There is nothing higher than life itself. The best enjoyment in the world is in life, not in the objects of the world. We worry a great deal about the world and about others, but do not have any awareness of what is happening within. We should be aware that there is something called misery accompanied by pain and that we are afraid of this misery. Refusal to accept that which opposes or upsets us leads to developing defense mechanisms. But by becoming observers of life, acceptance of its misery becomes possible. The problem starts when one does not accept pain, misery, problems, conflicts, or anything uncomfortable. One should learn to accept these things and then deal with them.

All the ancient scriptures and great men of the world teach how to attain that spirit of mind which is balanced and tranquil. Why should it not be possible to attain this level of understanding? If someone has done something in the past, someone can do it today; and if someone can do it today, then everyone can. But we need to systematize this knowledge. We must first understand and then apply those techniques which will help us attain this state of perfect health. Unfortunately our present-day models of health and therapeutics such as modern psychotherapy lack certain vital principles of holism. The holistic approach should be educational, teaching the participant methods to improve his own physical and emotional state. Holistic therapy should be individualized, equipping one with a comprehensive program which will allow him to grow, expand his awareness, and provide him with the strength needed to prevent him from slipping back into the grooves of his old habits. These skills must be self-learned and self-practiced. One should not have to depend on the therapist for motivation. It should come from within. As the participant perfects the methods of self-analysis, examination, self-control, and self-awareness, then he becomes more independent and better able to handle the day-to-day problems of life. Most importantly, he also learns how to transform his inner personality, and this will lead to a state of freedom from all pain and misery.

How does one go about attaining this state of health? The first step is to learn to accept that which makes one unhappy, for only then can he build a positive attitude. Learning to accept those aspects of the personality which cause unhappiness will lead to an understanding of the sources of misery. And it is only after this understanding and acceptance that one can begin to consciously make positive changes and reconstruct habits. The next step in freeing ourselves from pain and misery and attaining a tranquil mind is to never make rigid rules for ourselves without examining our physical and mental capacity. For example, one may make it a rule that he is not going to eat at night. That night he wakes with an unrelenting craving to eat. Although he has made a promise to himself, he finds that urge overpowering and finally gives in. He goes to the refrigerator and starts eating. He feels guilty about being weak-willed, and this further increases his appetite and his food intake. He wakes up the next morning feeling sick and disgusted with himself. He thinks he will never have the strength to resist his temptations, and therefore stops trying.

Rather than accept guilt and defeat, one should learn not to have unrealistic expectations of himself or of others. If one makes his program realistic, then he will be encouraged. If we set simple, realistic goals, then we will succeed. Our willpower will not be dissipated, and we can watch our progress every day. Dissipation of willpower is disastrous. The more the mind is dissipated, the more the willpower is weakened. A one-pointed mind creates a dynamic will. Without understanding one's own capacity, one starts expecting too much from others and even from one's own self. One should start by developing the ability to examine himself, for only then can he learn to be aware of his own capacity.

Next, one should have his own thoughts that are independent of culture and religion and from these he should develop a philosophy of life which is simple and direct. One should be flexible and adaptable, able to meet the demands of the moment. One should avoid being too rigid. Rigidity cuts off the spontaneous flow of memory, and that which one really knows cannot come forward. Actually, it is not difficult to know again that which is already known. If one wants to know, just know. If one doesn't resist, then he will know it. It is the barriers and resistances which keep one from realizing that which he already knows. Human beings do not actually need any enlightenment. Everyone says that they want to be enlightened, but wise people say, "No, you claim that you want enlightenment, but your thoughts and actions lead you toward hindrances. Remove those attachments and you are already enlightened." Between you and reality there stands a wall, and when we start examining that wall, we find that one of the stones of its foundation is the fear which is deep-rooted within. We should learn to be free of it, but for that learning we must not make any rigid rules for ourselves. There are countless laws which govern this human life and many of them as yet are unknown. For instance, ask any physicist why electrons move toward protons and why protons go toward the center and they cannot reply. They don't know. Yet as we begin to explore inwardly, uncovering what is already within, we will begin to see, experience, and understand the fundamental laws of nature. By delving further into ourselves, even the subtler laws will come into awareness. Then nothing will be impossible. The great sages who achieved special powers simply understood the more subtle laws of nature. Their abilities are not gifts; human life is the only gift. What the sages did was cultivate knowledge; then they gained control through a grasp of the subtle laws.

Each person should fix a plan for himself. Many people don't make any plans, and if they don't, they can accomplish nothing; they cannot develop their willpower. One should have a program for life and should work for that. That is how to build. To work endlessly for nothing is not growth, but if one works for something and has a program to think of for tomorrow, then life becomes a beautiful poem. There are many abilities at one's disposal which can be consciously cultivated to achieve freedom from all pains, miseries, diseases, and disorder. These are described in the ancient scriptures, but the idea of holistic health should not be buried in books. It should be brought into practical use in order to build a healthy society. This is possible and can be achieved by applying these truths in a systematic way. The process begins by gaining control over the laws governing our bodies. This is the first level of this knowledge.

2
Cleansing

T he ancient yoga manuscripts describe two sets of mechanisms in the human body—one for cleansing the body, the other for nourishing it. They work together in harmony, balancing each other. In explaining ways to make the body healthy, the yoga manuals first make one aware of those systems which are busy in cleansing the body: the lungs, pores, kidneys, and bowels. One should watch and see that the lungs expand rhythmically, that the pores are functioning properly, that the kidneys are operating normally, and that the bowels move regularly. One should try to understand his natural cleansing systems and learn to control and assist them, because if the cleansing systems are not functioning properly, the nourishing systems cannot do their work. The body will begin to break down. For instance, one cannot inhale unless one has exhaled first. If one has not moved one's bowels, if he has not expelled that waste, then he cannot enjoy eating his meal. Resistance and irregularity create disorders and dis-ease in the body, and if the body is in discomfort and disease, the mind also remains under stress and the nervous system in tension.

One doesn't have to be highly educated to understand

the nature of the body's systems. For instance, if one has
to move his bowels, it is obvious that delaying is not a good
thing.   And yet I have seen very educated people, even
doctors, who obstruct this cleansing process.   This is not
healthy. To build a healthy body one has to cultivate certain
habits which will cooperate with the natural processes of
the body.   One should not be lazy.   One should learn to
regulate his habits and learn to be consistent, mindful, and
moderate.

There are a few very simple exercises designed to
maintain the strength of the four excretory systems of the
body. Although all exercises mentioned in the manuals are
important, the most important ones described are those that
have to do with regulating the motion of the lungs. It is
important to understand why one should practice these
various breathing exercises for breathing is more important
than eating.   There are yoga manuals which are totally
devoted to the science of the breath, for proper regulation of
the breath is the basis of good health. The breath is the
bridge between body and mind. It is the subtle thermometer
which registers the conditions of both body and mind. The
breath is the source of life. One can live weeks without food,
days without water, but only minutes without breathing.
Proper breathing is the key to good health. Modern scientists
are only now beginning to understand the relationship of
breath control with body physiology. It has been demon-
strated that by practicing simple breathing exercises, one can
control the heart rate, skin temperature, digestive organs, and
other functions which were until recently thought to be

beyond the control of the conscious mind.   The yogis, however, have known and practiced these skills for thousands of years.

The breath is a vehicle for the energy called *prana*, and inhalation and exhalation constantly function like two caretakers in the City of Life. The exhalation expels the used up gases and the inhalation supplies the vital energy— energy and *prana* from the atmosphere. If one can regulate the motion of the lungs, he can protect himself from many diseases and maintain an even emotional balance. Alternate nostril breathing has been found very useful in dealing with nervous disorders and deep even breathing can help in re- laxing tension. Again, modern research has now verified this and people have been cured of hypertension, tension headaches, and anxiety states simply by learning to practice diaphragmatic breathing and relaxation. Therefore, just as one takes care of his diet, so he should take care of his breathing habits.

One should be aware of inhalation and exhalation and make sure that they are regulated properly, for this will clean the lungs. The ancients mention varieties of breathing techniques they experimented with and found useful in producing these effects.   These include *nadi shodanam, kapalabhati, bhastrika,* and many others.* Anyone can prac- tice the simpler breath awareness exercises, but the more advanced techniques, those using breath retention, should be practiced under the strict guidance of a competent teacher.

* For further information, see *Lectures on Yoga* by Swami Rama and *Science of Breath* by Swami Rama, *et al.*, Himalayan Institute publications.

One should start learning to regulate the breath by practicing diaphragmatic breathing. If one learns to use this method he will be able to control the motion of the lungs which work in the body like the fly-wheel of a machine. The diaphragm is a dome-shaped muscle located under the lungs. One inhales by contracting or pulling down the diaphragm. This downward pressure forces the abdomen outward and sucks air into the lungs. Relaxing the diaphragm allows it to float up to its original position. When this happens, the air is expelled. By properly regulating the movement of the diaphragm, one can induce a profound physical relaxation and a deep feeling of calmness. One can cool down an over-charged body, and turn off the internal stress response.

The habit of breathing in this way can be formed by paying attention to the diaphragmatic movement for a few days. One can easily observe this movement if he lies down on his back and places one hand on the chest and the other on the abdomen. He should begin breathing, trying to imagine that he is inhaling air into the abdomen and pelvic area. If this is properly done, the hand on the chest should not move, while the hand on the abdomen should rise with the inhalation and fall with the exhalation. This can also be practiced standing. Keeping the head, neck and trunk straight, one should place his hand on his abdomen and watch the movement of the diaphragm. He should gently push in and exhale; then let the abdomen come out and inhale. He should fill the lungs, but not overdo it. If one starts using the diaphragm to breathe, it will become a habit in ten days' time. Practice every day for a few minutes in the morning and the evening; it will help one to perfect a habit that will become a meaningful part of his life. Breathing diaphragmatically may be one of the most important of all conscious acts, as it is certain to produce a sense of tranquility, reduce stress and tension, adding years to one's life.

There are four basic things to watch for in learning to breathe properly. First, one should learn to fully fill the lungs with each breath. He should learn to breathe deeply; it is very simple if one is aware of what one is doing. In breathing deeply, one can use his full lung capacity, and slowly he will find that this capacity is increasing.

Secondly, as one practices breathing he should be sure that he is not creating a long pause between the inhalation and the exhalation. This is very important. One can form bad habits if he is not cautious and if he is not aware. For instance, a pause that takes any longer than the blink of an eye is a sign of a poor breathing system. At the Himalayan Institute research has been done to chart breathing patterns. It has been discovered that anyone who creates a long pause after expiration either already has certain symptoms of heart disease or is predisposed to the future development of coronary disease.

The third thing to observe in the breath is the regular flow of the inhalation and exhalation. The breath should be smooth. There should be no jerks in the breathing. If someone receives a mental or emotional shock, it will be recorded in the breath as a jerk. Thus emotional reaction can disturb the motion of the lungs and the pumping station of the heart. That, in turn, will disturb the vagus nerve and the rest of the

involuntary nervous system. When the breath flows smoothly, relaxation occurs; when it is irregular the body cannot
rest. By watching a baby deep in sleep and observing the
rhythmic motion of the abdomen, one can see how to perform proper breathing.

Lastly, one should watch for noisy breathing, which
is a sign of obstruction in the nostrils. The breath should be
silent, without turbulence. If done correctly, one will notice
a sensation of coolness at the tips of the nostrils upon inhalation, and a feeling of warmth on exhalation. If there is
an obstruction in the nostrils, and it is allowed to continue,
then one starts inhaling through the mouth, which is not
healthy as a normal practice.

Furthermore, there are some things that anatomy does
not teach us. One of these is that breathing through the left
nostril is different from breathing through the right nostril.
This is due to the tiny nerve endings at the base of the nose.
These nerve endings connect directly to the brain and are
stimulated by smell and also by the flow of the air as it
passes by. Thus air flowing through the left nostril will
cause nervous impulses to be sent to one part of the brain,
signalling restfulness and calmness, while when right nostril
breathing predominates the body is prepared for more active
processes such as digestion. It has been scientifically
accepted that if one of the nostrils remains continually
blocked, one will frequently experience pain and headaches.
What is more, when the discharge from both nostrils has been
examined, it has been discovered that they have different
electrical potentials—one being positive and the other being

negative.

Therefore, the nostrils are very sensitive and important anatomical structures and should be treated properly. They should be cleansed regularly, and there are various ways of doing this. One of them, called *neti kriya*, involves cleaning the nostrils by pouring lukewarm, saline water first through one nostril and then through the other, allowing it to flow out the opposite side. The practice also helps prevent colds, allergies, and hayfever. Another practice is called *sutra neti* or string cleansing. Here, a length of sterilized cotton cord, which has been blunted on one end by beeswax, is gently inserted into the nostril until it can be felt at the base of the tongue. Then one grasps this end, pulling it out through the mouth, gently moving the thread back and forth and then finally removing it, leaving the nasal passage clear. Both *kriyas* will clean out excessive mucus, open up blocked passages, and make breathing easier.

After one learns to breathe properly, he will find that his thinking has become very clear. When one learns to regulate his lungs by eliminating shallowness, pauses, jerks, and noise, then he has done his work as far as cleansing the lungs is concerned.

Regulation of the breath is essential for cleansing the lungs, but control of the breath can also be used to cleanse the pores. The yoga manuals describe many useful cleansing practices, among which are one hundred and eight kinds of baths—tub baths, herbal baths, sun baths—in fact, there are entire works devoted only to bathing. All these baths are external except one, and it is the finest of all. It is called the

prana bath. For this one doesn't expose himself to water, or
to sun; he just sits quietly. When one bathes with water, he
is not cleaning the pores. An external bath can only clean
the upper layers of skin. However, when one takes a steam
bath or sauna bath, the heat causes the pores to open and be
cleansed. The *prana* bath is similar, but the heat is generated
internally, with the help of willful breathing.

This cleansing of the pores with the help of breathing
should only be done by those advanced students who have
learned the method of breath retention. This exercise was
developed for those students who live in caves with the desire
of attaining *samadhi*. For them exposure to the sunlight is
immaterial. The *prana* bath is better than the sun bath or
any other bath. It is done in the accomplished posture with
the help of the abdominal lift, root and throat locks, and
inner retention. But it must be executed very carefully and
properly or the fine tissues of the lungs will be injured.
Ordinarily, the preliminary exercises of breathing described
earlier will be sufficient to help in cleaning the pores.

Bad odor and discoloration of the skin are symptoms
of ill health, and using deodorants and unnatural soaps and
lotions or medicines on the skin only hides or covers this
fact. By suppressing the natural means for ridding oneself
of these toxins in applying these deodorizers and other
chemicals, one is only asking for trouble in the future. The
extra burden of these toxins now must be taken over by the
kidneys, and this will cause an excessive strain on them. Man
was designed to sweat. There is a purpose and a reason for it
and by interfering with one's own cleaning system, one is

creating ill health.   Besides the *prana* bath, cleansing the pores can be accomplished by practicing certain advanced yoga practices such as the peacock, headstand, and bellows breathing. In fact, these provide an even better cleansing than can be accomplished by jogging or other forms of vigorous exercise.

There are certain specific cleansing exercises called *kriyas* which are described in the ancient manuals for cleaning the internal system.   These techniques leave one feeling refreshed and purified of excess mucus and other wastes, and they become as important as normal bathing to the regular practitioner.   This first is the upper wash, which is used to cleanse the stomach and bronchial passages. While squatting, one drinks about one and a half gallons of lukewarm salted water as rapidly and as steadily as possible and then throws it up.   This is done on an empty stomach and only juices are taken afterwards.   Another exercise, called *dhauti*, is designed to remove excess mucus from the esophagus and stomach.   It involves swallowing a three-inch strip of sterilized white cotton cloth which is about twenty feet long. The natural gag reflex helps remove the cloth and mucus rapidly.   These systems of cleansing may sound difficult at first, but once they are learned, they become easy.

To modern science mucus is considered only as a secretion of the internal organs.   However, to the yogis, mucus is not only a secretion necessary to line the delicate internal membranes, but also an excretion, a way the body rids itself of toxins.   Thus, excessive quantities of mucus production have always been considered by the ancients as a symptom of ill health. Many ailments of the lungs and stomach, such as asthma and certain types of indigestion have been helped simply by practicing these washes.

Just as the regulation of the lungs and pores is important, so is regulation of the bowels and kidneys. The kidneys are the toughest filters in the body, but they need natural cleansing every day. How can the kidneys be cleaned? The ancients found that the best natural agent to clean the kidneys is whey. I have experimented with this and I agree. Whey is the liquid which is left when one separates milk to make curds. When the milk is boiling, squeeze a lemon into it, and after it curdles, strain it. The clear liquid is the whey. Whey is not very tasty so one can use a little bit of honey in it if he likes. It should not be taken hot. Used regularly, whey is a very good diuretic.

Another way to cleanse the kidneys is to make sure to drink enough liquids. Don't misunderstand. This does not mean soda pop. All carbonated beverages and liquors are unhealthy because they irritate the intestines and leave deposits in the kidneys. I also avoid taking tap water because there are often many chemicals in it, and this too irritates the intestines and the kidneys. I take well water, but the well should be cleaned every year. Spring water is good too. Where I once lived, there was a hearty stream which I drank from, but when I came down to the city, I found the water packaged in bottles. No matter how wonderful water is, if it is kept bottled for prolonged periods, its properties change. They cannot last for a long time and so I don't recommend drinking bottled water.

The best natural liquids one can take are fresh fruit and vegetable juices. A glass of fresh orange juice, cucumber juice, or lemon water taken once in the morning, or twice if necessary, is very good for cleaning the kidneys. However, it should also be remembered that when one is thirsty, it is better to take pure water than to substitute with juices or bottled water.

Finally, the intestines too must be kept clean. For this, it is important to establish the habit of having a bowel movement the first thing every morning, and there is an ancient practice that will help one do this. Squeeze the juice of a normal-sized fresh lemon into a glass of water which has been boiled and add a pinch of mountain rock salt. This water should be warm, not hot, and sea salt should not be used because there is frequently sand mixed with it. Rock salt is crystallized and is much purer. The salt will draw out the waste material from the blood stream, but too much is not good. Only a little bit should be used. Adding honey to the water will give it a little taste so that it will be easier to drink and honey is very soothing for the intestines and good for the large colon. It is also a symbolic food. Only a bee knows how to make honey. It picks up the nectar from different places and converts it into honey. Those who are good students should be like the bee, picking up food and fragrances from different flowers and converting it into honey that is sweet to the mind and spirit.

After drinking the lemon water, one should squat down, feet apart, and place one hand on each knee. Then he should bring the knees to the floor, one after the other, beside the foot of the opposite leg. As one leg is pushed to the floor, the opposite leg is pressed against the abdomen, creating a slight pressure on the bowels. After doing this ten or fifteen times, one will feel like going to the bathroom. Drinking milk moderately every day is also very effective in emptying the bowels. Finally, if one stays on the toilet for more than five or ten minutes, there is something wrong. If he is just sitting there, thinking or reading, that is not good; it can cause hemorrhoids.

Fortunately, though, constipation is not a disease. It is caused by poor food habits, bad thinking, and a worried mind. If there is sufficient roughage in the diet, there will be no problem in regulating the bowel movement. Once one has had a bowel movement, one should not immediately rush for food.

The best sources of roughage are fruits, vegetables, and whole grains, not the bran that one buys at the health food store. Such bran is an irritant, though it may be quite effective in maintaining regularity. It is far better for one to obtain this roughage from whole natural foods, which contain gentler and milder forms of fiber.

Diarrhea, constipation, irregularity, and the poor functioning of the right vagus nerve (which helps digestion) can also be controlled by fasting. The Ayurvedic system says that fasting is very important for health and cleansing. But one should understand why he is fasting and should have a good reason. Some people fast for the wrong reasons, such as, "If you do not listen to me, I will fast," or "I don't feel good, I should fast," or "I just want to lose ten or fifteen pounds so I'll look good." These are not good reasons. Most people do this because they have been condemning themselves. They think that they are dirty; that they have done something bad. They have not washed those impressions from their minds and they think that by fasting, they will be able to do so.

One girl told me that she had been fasting for three months. She said, "I take only one meal." This is not fasting. If it were, then I have been fasting my whole life. Many people talk about total fasting. They do not eat or drink water when they fast. That is not healthy. There is no authority in the world that recommends total fasting. When one fasts, he should not take solids, but he should take liquids. He should take juices, like fresh orange juice, and water. He can also take some honey twice or thrice. But the finest thing to take is lemon, honey, and water. I have fasted many times, but I did it in a very systematic way. Fasting every week is dangerous. It deteriorates the natural resistance and makes the motion of the intestines and lungs irregular. Regulating the diet by understanding the value of the food one takes is much better than most of the fasting that people do. If the diet is good, one doesn't need to fast very often. Sometimes, on special occasions and under special circumstances, it can be helpful if done under the guidance of an expert who understands the nature of the body and the purpose of the fasting.

Here I would like to mention that those who like to do fasting for reducing weight do not achieve much. Controlling the habit of overeating is easy if one learns to supply that food which is needed by the body and particularly if one chews one's food properly. Dieting does not mean fasting. At most, fasting should be done only once a month. Nothing will happen to you then if you do not eat for one day. Every three months, when the season changes, fasting for three days in a row is very important, for many illnesses catch hold of you at that time because of the climate changes.

There are many more *kriyas* or methods of cleansing mentioned in the yoga manuals. Some of them, like *dhauti*, seem crude to modern men, but students who practice and want to arrest the untimely aging process find these practices very helpful. For them, experienced teachers recommend doing yoga cleansing exercises once every three months, with fasting.

3
Nourishing

Along with the cleansing techniques, the ancients stressed the importance of knowing about a balanced and nutritious diet. The body is our grossest tool and a very powerful instrument, and that which maintains the body is food. One should be practical and learn what type of food he should eat, how much food he should eat, and how much liquid he should drink. The quality of the food and the way in which it is prepared should also be understood. Yoga manuals talk about studying one's own capacity and regulating one's life accordingly. Neither overeating nor undereating are recommended. A yogi is one who knows his own capacity on all levels and regulates his diet and other activities appropriately.

There is no one diet that is perfect for all. Every person is different and unique. Each has a different metabolism; each requires different quantities of nutrients depending on his activity, his genetics, where he is living, and the state of his health. For example, an athlete requires much more food than a secretary, while someone who lives in the arctic will require more vitamin D in his diet than one living in the tropics. Likewise one who is recovering from a major illness, who is thin and undernourished, requires more nourishing foods such as milk and grains, while the person who has overeaten, or has polluted his body with cigarettes or drugs requires cleansers such as fruits. So the question of what to eat is an individual matter and each person must decide for himself what and how much to eat. However, there are some general guidelines that apply to almost everyone.

First, one should not become a victim of taste. The majority of modern-day people believe in taking tasty foods without concern for their nutritional value. But it does not necessarily follow that tasty food is healthy food, nor is it essential that all healthy food be tasty. All tastes are acquired just as other habits are. New tastes can be created by understanding that healthy food is helpful. Eating food should not become an unconscious habit like other addictions such as smoking or drinking.

One should watch carefully what and how he eats. Eating large amounts of artificially flavored, highly refined "junk" food is dangerous to one's health. Gulping down food and drink without proper chewing, or without resting between meals, or eating during stressful circumstances, leads to poor digestion. The stomach and liver will be overworked. Food will begin to ferment and putrify in the intestines. Thus food prepared and taken in such a way works like slow poisoning. One should start by choosing a diet that consists of unprocessed, unrefined, whole foods that do not contain artificial chemicals and by eating only when the body needs nourishment.

Unfortunately, few people follow this advice. As a

result of their poor food habits, many people have come to use unnatural methods to force themselves to do things which should come naturally. They take a cup of tea or glass of prune juice to go to the bathroom. To go to sleep, they take a pill. To digest food, they take a carbonated beverage. Instead of relaxing or regulating their breath to achieve a state of calm, they pick up their glasses and drink alcohol. In addition to this, the average person ordinarily takes more than one hundred twenty pounds of sugar every year. This is not needed. The several pounds of salt he eats a year is not needed either. Such abuse can be dangerous and even lethal. Medical research has shown that too much salt can result in high blood pressure and overtax the kidneys, and too much sugar can result in such diseases as obesity and diabetes.

On the other hand, the organic sugar in dates, honey, and fruit juices is very healthy if used in moderation. For unlike refined sugar, it is found with other nutrients in natural proportions. Nowhere in this world can one find sugar (or salt, for that matter) that is 99.9% pure except in the supermarkets. When prepared in this form, these products act more like drugs, and are even more refined than some medicines. If one eats a tablespoon of salt or a cup of sugar, he will soon notice the pharmacological effects. So the next rule is to avoid using excessive quantities of salt, sugar, and other stimulants.

Most people do not know what foods they really need. They do not have a sense of what to eat. They may have a sense of when they are hungry, but then they eat anything that is easily available, without thinking about the nutritional needs of their bodies. People may think they are taking a proper diet, but "proper" means that which is healthy, that which does not create interference as far as one's life is concerned, and most people do not know what this is. People should be conscious of this reality, for even if they have knowledge of foods, if they don't apply it properly, they will not enjoy good health. If they just had this little bit of knowledge, they would lead healthier lives and become more creative, helpful, and useful.

By practicing good nutrition, one can protect oneself from many illnesses, maintain sound health, and even create resistance to viral diseases.

As described in the ancient manuals, food falls into two different categories: cleansers and nourishers. Fruits have more cleansing value, while vegetables, grains, legumes, and dairy products have more nourishing value. One should include both types of foods in his diet every day. There should be a balance between solids and liquids. For most this means a diet that consists of about 40% whole grains, 20% beans, 20% vegetables, 15% fruits and raw vegetable salads, and 5% dairy products. During the winter one should eat less fruit because fruit makes one feel cooler. In the summer more fruit and raw vegetables should be taken and the quantity of whole grains should be reduced. In this way one maintains a proper balance.

However, some people favor extremes. They become food faddists and eat only raw foods, for example. Although it is very healthy to take some raw vegetables and fruit, not all the food that makes up a balanced diet can be taken this way. Beans may be impossible to digest unless cooked and certain vegetables contain harmful substances that are only removed by cooking. Many raw foods will irritate the linings of the intestines and cause diarrhea. In addition, the intestines, appendix, and liver are not able to digest large amounts of raw food. If someone were to try to live on dried fruit, for instance, his digestive mechanism would fail at some point and many undigested food particles, allowed to remain in the system for a long time, would ferment causing excessive gas, cramps, and other gastric and intestinal problems.

It is immaterial whether one is a vegetarian or not. I am not discussing "isms" here, but healthy food values. It is true, however, that the vegetable kingdom does supply sufficient nutritional content to offer all the necessary nutrients, and for those who want to lead a spiritual life, a vegetarian diet might be helpful. However, if one simply stops eating meat and substitutes poor quality foods such as candy, ice cream, or pastries, then this is not healthy either. If one wants to be a vegetarian one should be certain to eat only high-quality foods.

Sunflower seeds, almonds, soybeans, dried beans and peas (dahls) and some grains have sufficient protein. Indeed, some seeds and nuts are as rich as meat as far as protein is concerned. There are critics who say that even if a vegetarian eats the proper quantity of protein, he cannot get the best quality because there are very few non-animal proteins which are complete. This is true. The solution, however, is simply to combine a grain such as rice or wheat with a bean (dahl).

By doing this one creates a complete protein food that contains all the necessary amino acids in their correct ratio, without the harmful excesses of fat that are found in meats.

There are also other advantages to vegetarianism. People who are vegetarians are less likely to have constipation, hemorrhoids, high blood pressure, as well as certain kinds of cancer and heart problems. In addition, the effects of a vegetarian diet are noticeable in old people. Vegetarians have longevity of life and at the same time, in their old age they can normally think right, discuss things intelligently, and do their other duties. Many meat eaters, on the other hand, do not show such vitality in their later years. In the animal kingdom, carnivorous animals lack stamina and although they can fight fiercely, they cannot last for a long time. For instance, when the tiger and elephant fight, the tiger cannot last more than two and one half hours, but the elephant can fight for three days. The tiger is a carnivore and the elephant is a vegetarian. So it cannot be said that vegetarianism does not offer complete food value or have other benefits.

Whether one is vegetarian or non-vegetarian usually depends on his culture, but sometimes cultural habits also create problems in forming a healthy body. Such an unhealthy culture as ours needs modifications, but most human beings cling to their traditions and cultures so fanatically that they refuse to examine the cultural habits which may be making them unhealthy. Modern man calls himself civilized, but he suffers increasingly from degenerative diseases. What good is a civilization which makes one sick, weak, and incompetent?

In an attempt to slow this process of degeneration, people often turn to vitamins and other nutritional supplements. They often think that these aids will be a panacea for their ills. People often ask, "How many vitamins should I take?" The ancient manuals do not even mention vitamins. However, they do speak of vitalizers such as certain juices, herbs, and other natural foods. The juice of fresh vegetables and fruits contain a very large quantity of natural vitamins and minerals. Taking them one won't need to take artificial supplements. Vitamin C, for example, is readily available in the juice of fresh oranges and other fruits, and these vitalizers are easy to digest in this form.

However, if the fibers of fruits and vegetables are not properly ground and pressed, the organic value of the juice will not be fully extracted. In separating the juice from the fiber, one has to know how to crush the food properly so that the juice retains the unique property of that fruit or vegetable. Being in a hurry, people often use commercial juicing machines. These give them the juice, and they drink it and think that they have taken many vitamins in this way. But many of these machines are unsuitable and are not recommended, for many of the nutrients remain unavailable. The process that should be used is one that gently presses the organic juice from the ground fibers of vegetables or fruits. In this manner, all the vitamins are liberated. There are very few such machines for sale. However, no machine can be compared with the teeth since they have a powerful grip to chew the minutest fibers of food. So actually, chewing the fruits and vegetables is the best way of utilizing the properties that they contain. It should always be remembered that unchewed and unground food is not digestible, for the liver has no teeth.

Bad food and badly prepared food can affect all the nourishing organs of the body and disturb their functioning. Too many foods containing oils, for example, and too much "roasted and toasted" food or spicy food is unhealthy. It has frequently been observed that too much oily and greasy food can deteriorate the functioning of the nourishing organs. For instance, in the parts of the world where the people take in large amounts of fat and oil, many of them suffer on account of heart disease. Overcooked foods may also ultimately lead to ill health, so one should be careful about the food he eats, being cautious not to roast, toast, and bake it too much for the sake of taste. By doing so he changes the quality and also the chemical composition of the food, making it either indigestible or even harmful. Furthermore, it has no life, and, though it feels filling, it fails to fulfill the needs of the body. In such a situation, one may either overeat or loose his appetite.

However, if food is not cooked or crushed enough, it can also cause difficulties because it will not be easily digested or processed by the liver. One can compensate for this somewhat by chewing his food very thoroughly. The purpose in eating is not merely to get the bulk of the food, but rather to take the food value from the food. Therefore, the more one chews his food, the better it is for him. In addition, if one wants to lose weight, but doesn't want to curtail his meals, he should try this method: chew the food more and more and more—at least thirty five times. If one does this he cannot overeat, and he will lose weight easily. He is overeating because he is not chewing his food properly and is therefore not supplying the necessary food value to the body. In other words, the body needs something, and it is not being supplied, so the body is still demanding more food.

The best method for losing weight is to eat those foods which are suitable for one's own system. If the food is fresh and natural, selected and prepared properly, neither overcooked nor left undercooked, and if that food is chewed well, then one will not overeat or have a weight problem. Overeating is a very unhealthy situation and causes fat, one of the most powerful of diseases, which is also the source of many other diseases. The quantity that most people eat is more than they need, so one should watch his capacity when he eats and take a little bit less than his hunger requests.

Once one has a knowledge of food value and how to prepare food properly, he should learn how it should be eaten. It is very important to create a pleasant atmosphere before food is taken. One should not make haste or create tension before or while eating food. He should create a good mood while he is eating for even the scientists today know that food taken while one is upset will change into poison. This has something to do with the mind, the temperament, the endocrine system, and the body as a whole. After observing and collecting data from various homes, it was found that the food served on the table may have all the necessary nutrients but if the attitude prevailing while the family members were taking that food was not calm, or if they entered into

an unpleasant discussion, they later experienced such problems as indigestion, dispepsia, diarrhea, and constipation.
If a person is angry and distressed he will not be able to
create enough saliva and gastric juices. The stress, anxiety,
and anger affects the glandular system and its secretions.
Furthermore, under stress the intestines will become either
under or overactive, and this too will affect the whole digestive system. Food which has not been properly digested will
enter the large intestines and there the bacteria will convert it
into toxic or harmful substances. Therefore, the atmosphere
in which one takes food is as important as the food that one
takes.

One should never eat food, no matter how hungry he
is, if he is not cheerful. Don't poison the body by making
the dining table into a fighting ring. It is essential that one
creates a loving, pleasant attitude and atmosphere before he
eats. He should start some pleasant conversation, for example.
One's best friend, one's greatest physician, is the cheerfulness
that dwells within. So while taking food, one should learn to
be cheerful, for being cheerful is being creative. He should
not leave this in the hands of God by saying, "God make me
cheerful"; he must create it himself. Diversity is the essential nature of the universe, but cheerfulness is a human
creation.

The ancients always said grace before eating their
meals. This tradition has been part of all the great traditions.
This spiritual aspect of eating also has biological aspects: it
makes one calm and allows the gastric juices and saliva to
flow so that they can digest the food. It also helps to release

tension, which allows the intestines to work properly.   So saying grace or maintaining silence while relaxing and breathing deeply for a few moments before eating creates a state of harmony—a balance in the mind, body, and nervous system. Then when one eats he can relish his food. Food is not something to just be pushed in. Eating in a hurry is not healthy; it is, in fact, very dangerous.

After eating it is best to rest for at least five or ten minutes by lying on the left side. By doing this, the right nostril becomes active, supplying warmth and creating the necessary conditions for good digestion. This is very helpful. One can drink water half an hour after or half an hour before a meal, but drinking it while taking food is not recommended. It could be injurious to one's health for it tends to dilute and thus weaken the digestive juices. The ancients also say that it is dangerous to go to sleep right after eating. If one eats and then goes to sleep immediately, his digestion will not be completed and this will affect his circulation, heart, and autonomic nervous system, and he will have bad dreams. Why should one create a situation in which he might have nightmares?

In addition, snoring can be prevented by not overeating and by learning to breathe properly. People snore for two reasons: because they are overweight or tired. Also, one should be sure to wait for three or four hours after dinner before sexual activity because enough time should be given to allow the body to digest the food. If one engages in sex right after eating, then the blood supply will be diverted from the digestive organs to other parts of the body and digestion will be incomplete.

It is healthy to take juices, fruit, and other foods in small quantities several times a day rather than overeating or having a large, heavy meal at one time. For lack of time, many businessmen and busy people take dinner late in the day. It becomes heavy for the system and is not digested in time before sleeping. The evening meal should be very light. Midnight meals disturb the body.

Food taken at fixed hours also counts a lot. I collected data especially from bar attendants who work late at night and air hostesses who travel on international flights. Their digestive systems are always irregular and many of the host-esses reported to me that their menstrual period became irregular when they led an irregular life. Food and sleep influence the body. If food is taken on time, the system is regulated because of the regular habit. Irregularly taken meals during odd hours creates acidity in the system. Simi-larly there are countless other diseases which are acquired by irregular eaters.

If one takes these little precautions and practices these methods, he can avoid dyspepsia and other diseases and enjoy good health. These are the things that everyone should understand. They comprise the difference between human beings and animals. If a person has a dish before him, he can say, "I'm not eating; it is not healthy for me." If one's doctor says not to eat something, that person won't eat it, no matter how delicious the dish might be. But animals and young children cannot do this. They do not have enough sense or training.   Sensible people, on the other hand, understand when they are eating improperly or getting too attached to food, and then they change their patterns. The ancients cooked their food and ate it as an offering to God who created it for them, his instruments. It is important to remain healthy to be the instrument of the Lord and do one's duties selflessly. For those who understand the secret of life, their day-to-day life becomes an act of worship.

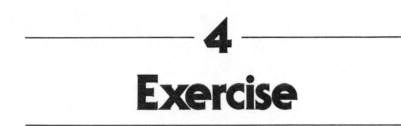

4
Exercise

The two different kinds of physical exercise essential to good health are stretching exercises such as the yoga postures and aerobic exercises such as jogging. Both are very beneficial for cleansing, relaxing and revitalizing the body and for helping it function properly.

Although quite different, they complement each other. The postures are relaxed, slow and gentle; they provide systematic stretching to all the muscles and joints of the body and massage the glands and organs. Aerobic exercise is active and stimulates the heart, lungs and muscles. Both kinds are necessary; each has unique effects which the other cannot produce. But they must be practiced regularly, carefully and in the correct manner in order to attain the desired effect. Doing either beyond one's capacity does more harm than good.

These days body therapies like massage, chiropractics, Rolfing, bioenergetics and reflexology are very popular. They all have specific benefits but are limited in two respects: one needs to rely on a therapist to provide the treatment, and the effects tend to be short-lived unless one returns again and again for more treatments. The yoga postures, on the other hand, are perfected gradually. This encourages self-reliance, and as one practices, observing his physical and emotional reactions, he will begin to notice definite positive changes in both body and mind.

An obvious effect of the postures comes from the stretch and stimulation they give to the muscles, ligaments and joints. This restores elasticity and tone to the body so that it eventually regains its natural shape. In addition, they stimulate circulation, revitalizing the internal viscera, the brain and the nervous system. The respiratory system performs more efficiently when one does the postures, for greater amounts of oxygen can then enter the system and more toxins can be eliminated. All the internal organs are massaged and toned, improving not only digestion but also bowel and kidney function. The endocrine system is stimulated and regulated to a fine balance. The postures increase resistance to fatigue and relieve tension. One learns how to relax, allowing the systems of the body to function properly. So the postures are a good, gentle tonic for the entire personality, making one feel healthy and full of energy. Excess weight is also reduced; the body becomes supple, and one moves with grace and ease. The complexion glows; the eyes shine.

By practicing the postures regularly, one gains control of the body and is able to maintain a steady, comfortable pose for increasingly greater lengths of time. One then begins to observe the finer functions of breath and mind, for only when the body is still can one turn within and begin to know oneself.

The basic goals of the yoga postures are to maintain a healthy body and gain peace of mind. Yoga texts tell us that many physical complaints come about in this way: a psychological disturbance can lead to a functional impairment which, in turn, is often reflected in irregularities in the breathing patterns. If this process continues, it can lead to actual cellular damage and manifest itself in a structural alteration. The yoga postures work first to correct the structural alteration and can be used as an effective therapy (particularly in the early stages) in reversing the above process. Then breath awareness and various breathing exercises can be useful in eliminating the irregularities which have developed in the breathing patterns. They can thereby help resolve the psychological disturbance which created the alteration in the first place. Thus, changes brought about through the practice of postures are not sudden or dramatic; they are deep and permanent.

At first the postures may seem awkward, but they have been systematically developed for centuries, through direct experience and observation, to calm, balance and regulate the systems of the body. When done properly and patiently at a regular time and place, one enjoys them, and they become a habit which brings a deep sense of calmness and much satisfaction.

There are over three thousand yoga postures, but only a few are basic. Among them are the cobra, boat, bow, plow, shoulderstand, fish, forward bend, spinal twist, headstand and stomach lift. The yogis lived close to nature and keenly observed their fellow creatures. Consequently, many of the postures (the cobra, locust, fish, scorpion, frog) are based on certain unique characteristics a particular animal displays. The postures are both natural and universal in nature and can be practiced by most people if they begin gradually, under the guidance of a competent teacher. It is not true that one cannot do them because it is not a part of his heritage. Anyone who wants to practice the postures can do so within his own capacity. But one should never strain or push for immediate results; doing so could cause injury and pain.

Practice in a quiet place, comfortably warm and free from drafts, where you can spread a blanket to lie on. Do the postures after bathing, in loose clothing. Stomach, bladder and bowels should be empty. Perform the postures systematically, with control and awareness, a calm mind and an attitude of respect. The mind remains passively alert and watchful; only those parts of the body needed to hold the pose should be tensed.

It is best to begin with some gentle warm-up stretches such as the joints and glands exercises. Start with the easier postures and work up to the more difficult ones. Most of the poses are complementary and should be done in a proper sequence with a short rest between each. Performing them in the morning prepares the body and mind for the activities of the day. Performing them at night soothes the nerves and helps one to relax. Since the body is more flexible at night, the postures are more easily done then, but morning practice sets a wonderful tone for the entire day. So fit them in according to your own schedule and temperament.

In addition to the postures, one can also practice dynamic, aerobic exercises, and jogging is very good for this. Jogging is popular nowadays, but there is much misunderstanding about the proper way to perform it, and many people have harmed themselves by doing it incorrectly. Some people force themselves, pushing and straining and trying to do too much too soon. One should always prepare oneself first and work within one's comfortable capacity. One should enjoy jogging; it should not be a form of self torture.

Jogging has been shown to be effective in reducing depression and major psychoses as well as in decreasing anxiety. It appears to be at least as effective as psychotherapy or tranquilizers with borderline schizophrenics, and it works as well as group psychotherapy with neurotics. It increases mental concentration and clarity, and it makes one alert and energetic. Those who jog are less affected by stressful situations than those who do not, and they respond to them less, physically and emotionally, because they do not secrete as many excitory hormones when under sudden shock or ongoing pressure. Those who jog sleep less than most and more soundly, and since they are not drowsy when they are awake, they do not need to rely on coffee, cigarettes or sleeping pills in order to work or relax. Jogging gives one a natural and healthy outlet for expressing the physiological reactions of the fight-or-flight response to threatening situations.

So much of modern life is full of stress that if you do not have a way to overcome the resulting tension or to express it beneficially, then you keep it inside. That can make you sick; it is one of the reasons people have ulcers, heart attacks, headaches and upsetting emotions. They do not know how to live in the world and yet remain centered and calm within, above the rush and roar of daily life. Jogging can definitely help you in this way, and it does this by making some specific changes in the body.

First of all, it helps your lungs operate more efficiently, strengthening the muscles around them, making them stronger, increasing their vital capacity, decreasing their residual volume and opening up previously unused space. Circulation is increased as the networks of blood vessels open up to nourish and cleanse the body. The heart is strengthened and toned, making it very healthy; in fact, it is actually enlarged, thus increasing its efficiency. The resting heart rate is decreased through jogging, as is the heart rate required for any given level of exertion. This happens because the heart pumps more blood with each stroke. It thus needs to beat less frequently, thereby conserving energy. Through jogging, the muscles increase in tone and strength so one can move with greater speed, endurance, flexibility and grace. Jogging burns calories (one hundred calories per mile), but more important, it resets the appetite mechanism in the brain, so one eats less and loses weight. In addition, less acid than usual is secreted in the stomachs of joggers, thus decreasing the possibility of ulcers. Jogging also acts as a natural cathartic so that the bowels of joggers are usually regular, and constipation is rare. Jogging also helps to normalize diabetes, hypoglycemia and other blood sugar problems. It purifies the entire system, aiding the elimination of wastes from the bowels, bladder, pores, mucus membranes, lungs and the cells themselves. Through jogging the pain threshold is modified so one can be less distracted by bodily discomfort. Thus, the whole body functions more smoothly and efficiently when one jogs, and the mind and emotions are calmed.

To begin jogging, it is best to dress warmly in absorbent clothes such as cotton sweatsuits, but any loose clothing will do. Keeping the body warm helps the cleansing process by increasing sweating. Any comfortable running shoe is good, but if one runs on the pavement the shoe should be well cushioned. Running on the earth is better, but extra caution must be taken to avoid stumbling and injuring oneself. Before jogging, it is very important to stretch the muscles and to practice some deep breathing exercises.

Jogging can be slow, regular and steady so you can go for a long time without tiring. Done this way, it is gentle but very effective, and it will not harm the body. Proper breathing for jogging is always diaphragmatic, and you should breathe through your nose, exhaling for twice as long as you inhale. Exhalations should be complete so all the toxins are eliminated from the system.

It is helpful to listen to the sound of the air going out over the soft palate and through the nostrils while you concentrate on exhaling completely. A good way to set the proper pace for jogging is by observing your need for air. If you cannot get enough breath through your nose, then you are going too fast and straining, and you should pull back. It is possible to go to almost your maximum capacity while you are still breathing through your nose, and if you feel that you cannot get enough air, you are exceeding your limit. If this happens, you should break your jog and walk until you catch your breath. You should jog comfortably at about three-quarters of your capacity.

Jogging on the balls of your feet is the best way to go for these slow jogs. This keeps the movement light and flowing and cushions the feet, ankles, shins, knees and hips, protecting them from injury due to a harsh impact. Landing on the toes also increases the massaging and stimulating effects of jogging.

Do not let your mouth hang open or your arms flop when you jog. Remember that you are breathing through your nose. Keep your lips together. Gently hold your arms up close to your chest, with your loose fists rotating about it as you move, and keep your elbows close to your body. Be sure to keep your shoulders relaxed and your head up. Keep your spine straight, your whole body relaxed, and let the abdomen move freely in and out as you breathe. Always jog with full concentration, particularly on the breathing, and enjoy the process. This will bring a feeling of clarity, peace and energy, for the muscles are relaxed, the oxygen in the lungs and bloodstream are flowing freely and the mind has calmed down. But this is not the same as meditation. In jogging the body is active, and so the mind is active, but in meditation both are still.

You should take care when you are jogging downhill, slowing down and landing gently so that you do not injure your knees or feet. Jogging itself should be rhythmic and natural. I have watched the faces of some joggers who look as if they were in agony as they pound down the street. This is not the way. The movement should be smooth and graceful. You should enjoy it, and you should always let up if you are in pain. Do not ignore the pain; learn from it so you can discover the proper way to jog. Experiment until you find a way that is not painful to you. Your body will direct you to the natural way if you do not force it. Be kind but disciplined, gentle but firm.

There are several variations to jogging that give one special benefits. A very good one is the twisting jog. Here, the torso and arms twist from side to side in rhythm with the pace. The arms create momentum as they swing, and the level at which the hands are held helps determine the point of the twist. This twisting and turning invigorates the spinal nerves and massages the viscera. Another variation is jogging with the arms raised high overhead with the hands folded. This lifts and expands the chest so that more fresh air can flow through the lungs, and it gives a good stretch to the arms, chest and abdomen. A third style is to lift the knees high and to kick the heels toward the buttocks as you jog. This helps the knee joints and results in more exertion.

When you have finished jogging, do not stop abruptly, but slow down gradually or you will stiffen. If you have been breathing properly, profuse sweating may occur, and this will cleanse the entire system. You should avoid taking a bath or shower until at least half an hour after jogging, however, because it may shock the system, and the pores should be given time to keep the sweat flowing. You should keep warm during this time.

It is good to stretch again after jogging to avoid cramps or sore muscles. The yoga postures are best for this. One can do them either before or after jogging, or both. Jogging after postures leaves one loose and stimulated; jogging before postures leaves one calm and balanced for the day. But if all you can do is jog, then do it. Do the postures at another time.

You will be more likely to jog regularly if you make it a part of your daily schedule. Then it becomes a habit which you accept and which the body automatically prepares for. In this way unconscious resistance is lessened. If you are obese, older or very out of shape you should begin by walking before you jog. You can get yourself started by taking the easiest step in that direction. Just stop what you are doing and go outside when it is time. If you do not want to change clothes, then jog in what you are already wearing. If you feel too tired to jog, then just walk, and soon you can pick up the pace. Often you will find that you are not as tired as you thought you were. But don't set rigid limits for yourself. If you have determined to go for fifteen mintues and feel too tired to continue after ten, then stop. Let your body guide you. You should gain energy from jogging, not lose it. Do not push, but also do not be lazy. After several weeks of daily practice, jogging will become a habit.

At dawn the air has a special quality, and it is very good to jog then. Late afternoon, when your energy may be low, is also a fine time to jog. Another good time is when you are already feeling low, because jogging will reset the metabolism and invigorate you. It is also hardest to get going then, so just form the habit, and it will be easier to do it. Never jog on a full stomach, however; let at least several hours go by after a meal.

Jogging out of doors is better than doing it inside, but jogging inside, or even jogging in place, is better than not doing it at all. Jogging twice a day is an excellent practice. It need not take longer than fifteen minutes to gain the benefits. One hundred breaths is a good run, and so is five hundred steps at a comfortable, loose pace. Three miles a day is a good goal to work toward. Long, fast jogs are not as effective as regularly practiced slower and shorter ones for attaining all the physical and emotional benefits possible.

In the early stages jogging may be difficult, since you cannot do as much as you would like to, but growth occurs in plateaus, and one day you will suddenly be able to do much more than you could before if you do not set your progress back by giving up or by pushing too much. Do not do either, for jogging is a powerful practice which creates overall well-being and a sound inner environment for spiritual development. It is the perfect complement to the yoga postures.

Women can do all of these exercises just as men can, but they should refrain from performing them during menstruation, the last five or six months of pregnancy and the first six weeks or so after delivery. Women should view the first few days of the menstrual cycle as an opportunity to rest and practice relaxation, diaphragmatic and alternate nostril breathing, meditation and inspirational reading rather than doing any strenuous exercise. The body is going through a natural cleansing process at this time, and it is not healthy to divert energy away from the places it is needed. This is not a sexist bias; it is a physiological reality. Practicing postures or jogging at this time could cause cramps and excess bleeding. Practiced at other times, however, the exercises create a strong and regular constitution which makes the so-called female problems less of a problem. Therefore, less discomfort and fewer irregularities are experienced during periods, and menstrual disorders are corrected.

Pregnancy and deliveries are also made easier if one has been practicing the postures regularly. Some simple standing, seated, squatting and reclining postures, which do not affect the abdomen, can be continued during menstruation, pregnancy and post partum adjustment, but the inverted, backward- and forward-bending postures are not recommended. The squatting posture can help decrease discomfort from cramps, however, during menstruation. After the fourth month of pregnancy women should cease all postures except for a few simple stretching exercises. Any postures involving the pelvic area can be dangerous to the unborn child. Women who want to begin the yoga postures for the first time should wait until six months after delivery to start.

The most beneficial posture for an expectant mother is the relaxation pose which should be practiced extensively along with diaphragmatic breathing. Pregnant women should not jog at all, but regular walking is very good. When jogging, women should protect their breasts, wearing garments that support them firmly or holding them still by folding their arms underneath them. Women should be especially careful to jog on the balls of their feet in order to land gently and prevent displacement of the uterus. Jogging seems to be an especially beneficial practice for women since they seem to be prone to the complaints it corrects and also because they frequently do not engage in other forms of physical activity.

Children are naturally flexible and eager to play, stretch and run. They enjoy their bodies and love to learn new ways to experience them. In a household where the yoga postures and jogging are practiced, the children will pick them up by watching their parents. Otherwise, they can be taught a simple program of postures by age seven or nine. But since they have shorter attention spans and lack the muscle strength and control of adults, the length of time they hold the postures should be shorter, and they should not be forced to go beyond their limitations. Care should be taken in teaching the inverted postures to children, since their bones and muscles are not fully developed and they cannot safely support their own weight. Prolonged practice of the shoulderstand is not advised for pre-pubescents because of its stimulating effects on the thyroid gland which regulates growth. Children under twelve can perform the cobra, half locust, bow, forward bend, plow and *yoga mudra* without harm, but it would be best to avoid the headstand, peacock, stomach lift and other difficult practices until age twelve or puberty. Adolescence is a good time to begin the practice of the yoga postures, but it is not so essential in childhood.

Jogging is very good for children. Although they

generally run and play a great deal, a surprising number are not in good shape because they do not take part in regular exercise. Jogging gives them a good way to do this. It also helps them release built-up energy and provides a chance for the entire family to do something together. Jogging is good for the child who is not very skillful at team sports or dislikes competition. It is a healthy activity and can help him feel better about himself at the same time. Children should be careful, however, not to overexert themselves or exercise without paying attention to their motions.

These exercises will give children strength, endurance, agility and coordination as well as prevent many diseases while improving their state of mind. It has also been found that the IQ of a child can be increased by enlarging his intake of oxygen through correct deep breathing, and breathing is improved by both postures and jogging. Good habits formed in childhood shape the life of the adult to be.

Advanced age, however, is not a barrier to beginning, or practicing, the yoga postures if it is done with care. It is never too late to begin, or resume, these exercises, and their benefits are always available. The postures are beginning to be taught in nursing homes, and the elderly enjoy practicing them gently and experiencing their effects.

Older people need not merely await degeneration and death. They can use their time to become healthier than they ever were, but they should begin with gentle stretching exercises, and they should always be careful not to extend beyond their comfortable capacity. They can benefit a great deal from the yoga postures since their effects decrease some common ailments of old age: hypertension, stroke, diabetes, insomnia, arthritis, digestive disorders, constipation and chronic aches and pains. Stiff joints, brittle bones and fragile ligaments and muscles should be protected by cautious awareness, but within these limits the elderly can increase their enjoyment of life with a program of these stretches.

The same is true of jogging if one begins gradually, with a regular program of daily walking. The pace can eventually become faster and the distance longer until it is comfortable to do a slow jog once or twice a day. This is very good for regulating and rejuvenating the entire system. Weak and infirm people in nursing homes have become healthy, lively and happy because they have taken up exercise programs consisting of jogging and postures. The quality of their lives can definitely be improved so that they look forward to surviving longer. Illness often follows inactivity and depression, but it can be removed with exercise and a sense of purpose and well-being. There are many marathon runners who are in their sixties and seventies. Age is no excuse to avoid taking responsibility for one's health.

A measure of vitality, awareness and peace is thus available to all who seek it, and a good way to start is to get the body in a healthy condition through exercise. Only when one is healthy and strong can the mind, will and emotions be trained, and this is essential for spiritual growth.

5
Being Still

It is only after one has learned to take care of the body that one can tread the path of inner life. Proper cleansing, nourishing and exercise are the prerequisites for the next step in the cultivation of health. This step is called being still. It is very important and, if one studies it systematically, not very difficult. Once one has prepared the body, it is essential that he learn to sit quietly. Even if one eats the best diet, if he does not know how to be still, his mind will not yet be under his control. The most magnificent sports car, if it is driven recklessly, will soon be destroyed. So it is with the human being. A strong body willed by a reckless mind leads to restlessness and ill health. One should become aware of the integration of the mind and body for the mind and body have such a close relationship that the body can disturb the mind. If the body is in a state of pain or disease, then the mind will also be ill at ease. Likewise, a restless mind creates a tense and nervous body.

It should be remembered, however, that in general the mind rules the body. The mind moves first, and then the body follows so one's body language is totally dependent on his mental functions. Try this and see. Try to raise your arm without first thinking about it. It cannot be done. In order to raise the arm, one must first think, "Arm raise," and then send this message through the nervous system from the brain to the arm. The arm will not move until the mind tells it to do so.

Furthermore, just as the mind sends messages to the body, the body is continually sending messages to the mind. "This chair is hard, this posture causes a pain in the back." When the mind is constantly being badgered by all these body messages, it becomes very active, agitated, and dissipated trying to integrate all the data. It cannot remain calm.

Therefore, in order to learn to be still, one must first quiet the chatter coming from the body. This begins by learning the art of sitting. By developing a steady, comfortable position, one frees himself from the distractions of the body and is able to attend to the mind. For if one's body is not steady, his mind cannot be still, and if one puts the body into an uncomfortable position, it will become a constant source of distraction. In addition, if one sits in a certain position for a week and then changes to another position the next week, one's mental attitude will change as well. So choosing a position in which one can be still is very important.

The Bible talks about the importance of stillness. "Be still and know that I am God." If a human being learns this, then that godly part in him will reveal itself. But for that godly part to be revealed without being still is not possible. So one should direct one's voluntary and conscious effort to learning how to be still. If one just learns this there will be no problem. In the beginning, this means not moving at all, but later, once one learns what stillness is, one will be able to move the body, to act and live in the world, yet remain still. Calmness, stillness, and a one-pointed mind are identical and when this is realized, it becomes possible to create them at all times.   In other words, true stillness does not merely mean the absence of movement. It means having equanimity and then performing one's own actions responsibly. It means attending effortlessly to one's duties without being affected or being "bent out of shape" by the external circumstances.

To achieve this goal requires first of all self-discipline. Whereas all the activities of animals are governed by nature, that is not the case with human beings. Human actions are governed by one's desires and these can be controlled only through self-discipline.

Many people are afraid of the word "discipline," for discipline when imposed by others is definitely frightening. But self-accepted discipline helps keep the body healthy and the mind sound.   Discipline really means regulating habits, and habits are the basis of human character. One spends his whole life identifying with one's personality, with this character, but who built it? God? Nature? No. One's own habits have woven a character for him, and their pattern makes up his personality. One's habits are deep-rooted in motivation.   One can strengthen these habits or one can change them. If one really wants to change and understands how habits are formed, then he will come to know that there are simple practices for doing this. With time, and with the help of these laws, one can systematically bring about that inner transformation which is called *samyama* in the ancient texts. One cannot change one's face or other external forms and shapes but he can completely transform his internal states. Today one might condemn and feel bad about oneself because of one's habits, but tomorrow he can completely transform himself and come in touch with his inner potentials for creativity, happiness, and truth.

Self-discipline can only be achieved through the conscious directing of one's will. Will is a very powerful tool for making one successful, and willpower is created by a one-pointed and concentrated mind. The more one's mind is dissipated, the more willpower weakens. It is not easy to control the totality of the mind, for the mind is very vast. In fact, the ancient scriptures say, "Vastest of all is the mind." There is only one thing that is vaster than the mind and that is the center of consciousness. But that portion of the mind which we use in our daily lives can be brought under control very easily if one learns and practices a systematic approach.

The first thing to learn is regularity, or consistency in one's practice. To do this one should form the habit of sitting quietly once or twice every day. For learning to be still it is important to find a comfortable and steady pose, either on a chair or on the floor. Steadiness comes when one keeps the head, neck, and trunk in a straight line. For a few days, this might create a little bit of uneasiness, but gradual and gentle practice will help one in sitting steadily and comfortably. Again, overdoing this is not at all recommended. It is better to sit correctly for five minutes twice a day than to sit once a week for an hour.

In trying to find a position in which to sit, many people who have read Eastern books begin with difficult postures, such as *padmasana* and *siddhasana*, (the lotus and accomplished postures) without first making their bodies supple. By doing this, one can strain the knees and cause pain, discomfort, and even physical injury. One will be disturbed by the discomfort and will not achieve stillness. Instead of doing this, he should sit in any easy pose that makes him comfortable and straight. Then he can learn to be physically steady. It is important to keep the head, neck, and trunk straight because if one is sitting crooked or is slumping over, he is not allowing the spinal cord to be aligned correctly. Then the three sensitive channels there—the central canal in the middle, and the sympathetic and parasympathetic cords on either side—cannot function properly. When the body is still, one should not be tense. Any tension will be reflected in one's muscles and nervous system. One's whole body structure, the way he is sitting, forms a steadiness for him.

Practicing one posture every day at the same time is very important. So one should practice a posture in which he is comfortable and steady. One posture that should not be used for this process is the corpse pose. This pose, done by lying on the back with the legs and hands at the sides slightly away from the body, does induce deep relaxation and is very comfortable, but it is not considered steady. By practicing this pose, however, one can learn to ease physical tension.

Releasing physical tension is very important because muscle tension can create havoc in our body, affecting the heart, brain, liver, and digestive system. In learning to relax, one should lie down on the back with the legs about eighteen inches apart, the hands on the abdomen and, if the surface is hard, a soft pillow cushioning the head. Then one should systematically survey the body from head to toe and back, locating the tension points and mentally releasing them. Once one understands his own mental capacity, he will be able to be successful in doing this within a few days' time. It is very important that one not use auto-suggestion but rather that he observe the movement of the diaphragm and then breathe gently and deeply according to his comfortable capacity. Making the body still and then making the flow of the breath serene and deep will help in relaxing the nervous system and releasing the tension from the set of muscles that is governed by the autonomic nervous system. This relaxation exercise should not be practiced for more than ten minutes or one might fall asleep. After five minutes, one should voluntarily create tension all over the body, release it, survey the body again, and watch the slow, deep flow of the breath.

By practicing this exercise regularly, one will reap many benefits. Blood pressure will be lowered; the heart, liver, and digestive organs will function more effectively. One will have less tension, more strength and energy, and greater vitality. Simply by doing the corpse posture along with deep abdominal breathing increases longevity and fosters health.

One final reminder regarding regularity is that one should choose a specific time and consistently use that time to practice sitting. The best time is either early in the morning or in the evening. However, any time is fine as long as one will not be bothered by other duties, interruptions, or distractions. Regulating one's habits by being punctual in practice is important because it is necessary to counteract the pressure of bad habits which keep the body under stress. A body which remains constantly under the influence of such habits will always be unhealthy.

The second point to understand and observe in learning to be still is that it is necessary to cultivate patience with oneself. Suppose one wants to sit calmly but since he has never learned to do this, he can only sit for two minutes before his mind starts jumping about. He changes his posture, tries again to be still, then changes his posture again. One should accept this. Failure is the pillar of success, provided one takes advantage of the situation and learns from it. One should observe his capacity and go slowly. The first day two minutes is sufficient. It is said in the scriptures that if one can sit still, straight, and comfortably with a perfectly one-pointed mind for just ten minutes, he can attain *samadhi*. So it is best to increase one's capacity slowly and gradually and to learn to be patient with oneself.

Patience is a great virtue, but what does it mean? It does not mean being lazy nor does it mean an absence of effort or the failure to plan ahead. Being patient means being observant. Once one learns to be patient he will not condemn himself for problems with his thinking process. Patience is like standing on the bank of the river of life just waiting for one's ship to return. There is a flow. One does not repeat that which is done; he does not see that which is not yet done. He is patiently waiting to see the fruits of his deeds, being content with doing his best and thus making wise decisions for the future.

So one should learn to be patient with himself. You know yourself better than anybody else. That part of your personality which has never been exposed to others, you yourself know, for one always remains in touch with that part of himself which is not pleasant. Many people start identifying themselves with that part of their personalities and start condemning themselves. They do something one day, and the next day start condemning themselves for it. If the world does not praise them, if people do not appreciate them, they blame themselves. They are not aware of the innate source of strength within themselves. They should learn to appreciate and admire that part in them which is helping them, leading them. No matter how much they condemn themselves, no matter how bad they think they are, and even if the whole world says they are bad, still there are certain qualities in them which are very special and which make them unique. They should learn to admire those parts.

If the first step in developing stillness is making it into a daily habit, and the second is being patient with oneself, then the third is practicing constant observation. One should learn to observe his capacity. Although one may like to practice sitting, sometimes in the beginning of developing this habit, the mind will say, "What am I doing? This is silly. Nobody in our culture does this. Why should I be still? This is a foolish idea. Why don't I just get up and have a Coke?" But no matter what culture or religion one comes from, he should learn to be still for the sake of his health.

If one really follows these principles, there will be no problem. One should understand from the very beginning that stillness is essential because one cannot attain meditation until he can be still. Whenever one is attentive, he has to be still. This is the principle: one cannot examine an object when it is moving.

Physical stillness, however, does not mean mental stillness. When one learns to still the body, something else becomes more active. To make one's body still means to make his mind active, and when finally one begins calming down his conscious mind, he finds that the unconscious mind is activated, rushing in with memories, thoughts, and feelings, many of which were previously suppressed.

In the process of meditation, one first contacts the conscious part of his mind and learns of body-mind interaction. The conscious mind is that which one uses in his daily life during the waking state. By sitting in a particular place, using the same posture, holding the head, neck, and trunk straight, observing one's thoughts as they emerge, one is slowly able to begin to contact and calm the conscious mind and body. At this stage, one should pay attention to the body tremors and muscle tension, consciously releasing any muscular tightness that is perceived. Later, as the conscious mind and the body begin to rest, the unconscious mind becomes active and emerges into awareness.

In the beginning, one should not overdo this. It is his ambitious mind that says that he should try to do it for a long time, that he can sit for half an hour. This is a waste of time. Looking at one's watch to see how many minutes one has practiced is not helpful. One shouldn't try to show that he is a great yogi. One has to be great from within. Gradually, in a few months if one practices, he can learn to be still for a longer time, but there is no use in wasting time absent-mindedly daydreaming and hallucinating various images and calling it meditation.

When one sits to meditate, his memory becomes more active. He recalls what he has done in his past, who has been good to him, who has been bad to him, who has been his friend, who has been his enemy. Sometimes the unconscious brings forward one of the impressions from the bed of his memory that makes him either happy or unhappy, and he forgets that he is sitting for meditation, allowing himself to be completely carried away by that thought form. Involvement with thought forms in this way is not meditating; it is daydreaming. It is a waste of energy because it actually strengthens that part of the mind that is uncontrolled. So in order to learn the process of being still, one must gain control over the conscious mind.

At first, when the mind is flying here and there, it will be very helpful to practice breath awareness. This is very important, for the breath is very closely related to the conscious mind. They are interdependent. When the breath stops, the conscious mind fails, and that is called death. One can train and regulate the mind by being aware of his breathing, for breathing is the lamp that lights the path to increased awareness. By simply learning to observe the breathing process, one can reach a deep state of meditation. However, the first few days this will be an obstacle because one is trying to bring his conscious mind under control, whereas previously it had been controlling him.   It will resist and will not want to listen. As one starts to control it, however, it will change completely. When one first begins, he may notice while inhaling that suddenly the inhalation breaks and he feels as if he is suffocating or isn't able to catch his breath. One should continue to pay attention to the breath and nothing else and shortly this feeling will disappear. Let the mind be aware of the breath and watch how it flows. If one can do this for three minutes, only three minutes without any diversion, it will bring good results.

Besides observing the breath, one should also be aware of the sensitivity of the nervous system. Some people mistake sensitivity for psychic ability, but that is an error. I once had an experience that illustrates this point:

When I was a child living in Kalipur on the border between Tibet and India, I studied Kung Fu. I had been taught not to harm, hurt, or kill anyone, and I became very passive because I did not understand the principle of non-violence properly. If an animal charged me, I would not defend myself. So I was sent to a Kung Fu teacher who was over ninety years old. This old man had been blind from birth, but if I moved my finger in a circle, he would say, "You are making a circle." If I shook it, he would say, "Now you are shaking your finger." I suspected that he could really see and that he knew some trick to make himself appear blind, but when I asked him how he could do these things and told him of my suspicion, he showed me his empty eye sockets. I was amazed, but even then I thought, "There is some trick here. He knows how to turn his eyeballs in a different way." I was that skeptical.

One day he said, "Come over here. I am going to show you that I see everything not through my eyes, but through my sensitivity. I want ten of you to come at me with sticks and try your best to hit me. I won't have a stick myself."

I said, "I won't do it because you are a blind man."

He said, "You are taking useless pity on me for being blind. I am not. My nervous system is so active and sensitive that I can perceive any sound vibrations that happen near me better than you can. I can see things through my nervous system. I don't need eyes."

Then some of the students who knew him well started to attack him. He was in the center of a circle of ten people and quietly went through a gap in the circle, leaving the students hitting each other. He started laughing and said, "Do it again."

The second time, he snatched somebody's stick and started fighting with everybody. Nobody could hurt him. He was so sensitive to the things going on around him that he checked any move that was made. Through discipline and will, this man had developed his nervous sensitivity to a very high degree. He was able to see without sight.

Normally when someone looks at something, the sensation is carried by the optic nerve to the brain and then is distributed to the related parts of the body. The nervous system lies between the brain and the body. The body is actually like a house in which the nervous system is a large network of wires. The brain is like a bulb and the mind is the energy which constantly flows through that network which is the nervous system. If the house is not properly looked after, all its inner properties will be of no use. Also, if one has a wonderful mind and the bulb is broken, then too electricity will not be used properly. Similarly, if the bulb is very good and the electricity is flowing properly but the wires are cut at different places, then it will be of no use either.

All living creatures possess a nervous system, but each differs in its degree of sensitivity. For example, if a plant is cut, tears do not flow down its leaves. Though it has a nervous system of sorts, it is not very evolved. If some person cuts or hurts his foot, however, he will cry immediately, and tears will roll down from his eyes. He has an active nervous system. Nervous sensitivity is not just a physical trait. It is also a mental and emotional one. This actively working nervous system in human beings is a gift in the cycle of evolution and we should take advantage of it by developing it properly.

Many people are insensitive in their relationships because they don't understand how to cultivate the sensitivity within them. But one's emotional life is totally dependent on this sensitivity because sensitivity is part of awareness. Many times when people talk, they say, "I am aware of this." They are talking about certain facts, about being aware of something physical, something quite obvious.

Yet despite being sensitive to these external or superficial matters, many people remain oblivious to what is happening within. This changes when one begins to meditate.

During the early stages of meditation one can become very aware and very sensitive to the things he has done in the past and may feel guilty or unhappy about them. Rather than accept these feelings, most people resist them, for they do not know how to forgive themselves. They blame themselves. They have formed this habit and apply it to others too. So if somebody has done something which they don't like, they don't forgive them either. Gradually they have made themselves insensitive to the positive things in themselves and in others. They see only the negative. One should learn to forgive by doing it occasionally whether it is contrary to his desires or not. If one has committed a mistake, he should accept the fact that a mistake is only a mistake. He should not repeat it, but should not condemn his personality for it. In this way he can increase his ability to be sensitive.

If one does not appreciate and accept himself, it is because he has been doing negative meditation. This has made him what he is today. Worry is one form of negative meditation and it can become a deep-seated unconscious habit. One can create many diseases through his own mind and one can heal himself through this same mind. So one should learn to give himself positive feedback. "I am all right, and the life force is here in me. Why am I condemning myself? Why am I hurting myself?"

That mind which has the power to create guilt feelings and many diseases also has the power to heal, for it is completely controlled by the thinking process. Just learn that the mind is creating diseases and try to heal them instead.

Meditation is very powerful and therapeutic. There

could not be anything more powerful than meditation. I learned this lesson once when I was a boy. I fell down the mountainside and injured my right knee. A large, persistent lump developed there. One of the *swamis* said, "You can dissolve that lump with your mind."

I said, "I don't want that lump and yet it is still there."

He said, "You don't want yourself to be a bad boy and yet you are a bad boy. What do you mean by 'want'? Want is not powerful. You want yourself to be good and still you are not. You want that lump to dissolve and still it does not. So wanting has nothing to do with it. Learn to meditate. In meditation a one-pointed mind is developed and this creates a dynamic will. Willpower is a greater and deeper strength than wanting."

I told him, "You do meditation. If you think your mind is very powerful then why don't you just help me and dissolve this lump?"

He agreed and said that he would. He told me to sit down at such and such a time and in one week the lump would be gone. He said, "I could dissolve it right now, but I want you to become aware of the process and learn." In exactly one week the lump disappeared. I could not find a trace of it.

The first principle of learning to be still is regular practice; the second is patience; the third is observation; and the fourth is analysis. It is true that one must understand himself from within to attain a state of perfection, but analysis is not sufficient to transform the personality. After analysis comes the discrimination to make a proper decision.

One should never determine to do something unless he has explored all the consequences and chosen the best alternative for his development. This principle of choosing the best alternative is called discrimination, and is the fifth principle for developing control of the mind. The reason one experiences failure is because he does not know how to make decisions at the right time and place. His faculty of discrimination cannot decide in time because there is no strength behind it. One Urdu poem says, "When I was young I had strength, but I had no wisdom. Now that I am old, I have wisdom, but no strength." When one does not know how to decide things in time, there is a misuse of strength and a lack of wisdom. He cannot decide things in time because he has no determination, no willpower, and no understanding of one-pointedness. All success in the external and internal world depends on these factors. Therefore, as one progresses from one step to another it is very important to understand the mind and how it functions, for it functions in exactly the way one wants it to. The day one understands this and determines to change it, it changes of its own course. So one must understand one more principle—determination.

Once you have analyzed and decided what to do, then you should determine to carry it out. Determination is the sixth principle, but it should not be confused with obstinacy. Determination expands, but obstinacy contracts. Determination is slowly and gradually built by the willpower of a one-pointed mind. Developing willpower is like letting an internal earning grow. Just as one earns money, puts it in savings and is called rich when the interest mounts, so one should let his mind become rich from the willpower within him. One's willpower is at his disposal if his mind is one-pointed and concentrated. The more dissipation one has, the less willpower he has, and a dissipated mind is a constant source of stress.

Developing the skills of one-pointedness and determination is very simple, and one doesn't have to sit down and meditate to learn them. One can practice them while completing the activities of his everyday life. All he has to do is understand one thing: whenever he does anything, he should do it with full attention. No matter what he does, he should pay attention to it. For when one pays attention, he will find that he has improved his concentration, or one-pointedness. No matter how many *mantras* you have, no matter how many *gurus* you claim, you will never learn meditation by just sitting in a corner for fifteen minutes and then remaining uncontrolled the rest of the day. Doing something half-heartedly means that one is distracted. We must learn to pay full attention to what we are doing all of the time. This is a sign of growth. Paying full attention will make one aware of the quality of his work. Then, later, he can analyze it, "I have done this much, but to raise the fruits of my actions properly, I should have done more." All mental powers such as psychic powers, mind control, voluntary control, getting a hunch, and going to the source of intuition depend upon one faculty—the faculty of determination. With this strength, one can work with himself to create physical, mental, and spiritual health.

When one learns to become a self-healer, to think positively, he can progress. When one starts dealing with his mind and giving it an object to focus upon, this focusing of mind is called concentration. When one has developed the ability to focus the mind, then he learns to expand that ability, and this is called meditation. Without the expansion of individual consciousness, the individual does not grow but remains within the boundaries which he has built with his petty desires and narrow-mindedness. Expansion is a law of life, and to go against it is to create more ignorance for oneself.

When one one has analyzed the situation, decided what to do and determined to do it, then he should take action. If he does that, he will not fail; but if he does not take that final step even when he knows what to do and how to do it, then he has not succeeded. Knowledge means that one knows what to do, knows how to do it, and takes action in time. There is a Sanskrit word, *apta*, which means, " he who does and says whatever he thinks." Thinking, saying, and doing are the same for him. If one does not act, then he is not experimenting on what he has analyzed and decided in his thinking process, and this means that he is not wholly confident. If one is not confident, he cannot be self-reliant, for self-reliance comes when one has performed action. Then, and only then, can one weigh his own capacity.

Through meditation one can control that part of the mind which he uses in daily life. When one's consciousness starts moving upward he becomes aware of another level of life, and he understands more and more. A person who does not meditate does not know how to expand his consciousness. He has narrow vision as if he is looking through a window, but when he learns to expand his consciousness, it is like going through a door. It is exactly as if one were looking through a small window in a house. From the window his view is very limited, but when he goes out of the house, he has a much wider view. When he goes to the roof, he can see even more clearly. By the same token, as one's consciousness expands, his vision becomes clearer, and he understands things as they are. In *samadhi*, the individual learns to expand his consciousness, fathom all boundaries, and unite himself with the cosmic consciousness.

So through regular practice, patience, observation, analysis, discrimination, determination, and proper action, the mind becomes concentrated, and a concentrated mind can meditate very nicely. At last one reaches the state of *samadhi*, the state of tranquility in which he does things yet remains above them. Nothing can affect him. Then, as his consciousness goes to the height of *samadhi*, his wisdom increases more and more until complete transformation to a state of perfection takes place. This is the state of perfect stillness.

6

Emotions

People frequently talk about knowing the mind and its various faculties, but they don't talk about feeling. How can one know something without feeling it? When one perceives something, the first thing he is aware of is sensation. If one is not feeling something, he cannot know it, and if one loses the power to feel, he becomes insensitive. Those who are insensitive, who are not very emotional, who have learned to intellectualize everything cannot become creative. They do not realize that beneath the thinking process lies the real source of creativity, which is emotion.

The right use of thinking is expression, but the right use of emotion is creativity. Emotion is a very great power; it is the highest power in one's possession. When it comes to emotion, all human beings are one and the same because intelligence has no place before it. When one becomes emotional, he finds that his reason has left him and that he cannot help himself. When one is emotionally upset, he becomes blind, loses the power of discrimination, and his entire behavior—mind, action, and speech—becomes abnormal. Misuse of emotion is destructive, but this does not mean that all emotional power in itself is destructive. Those who are very emotional can become very creative if their emotions are properly guided and if they learn to direct them in a constructive way. People who know how to use their emotions creatively become successful in the external world and remain happy.

When emotion is led by devotion it is called ecstasy. The greatest things in the world have been done by people at the height of ecstasy. This is the work of emotion, not of the mind. The intellectual gymnasium is not helpful in knowing one's internal states. Though the mind is a very essential and powerful tool, it contains nothing new or original. It can only serve as far as the world of facts is concerned. Creativity and discovery lie beyond the mind. Emotion is the bridge between consciousness and creative thought. So one should learn to use the power of emotion to go beyond the limitations of thought.

Among the various functions of the mind, the intellect seems to be the finest, but without the help of emotional power, the intellect is like a lame man who is not capable of reaching his destination. Even the highest of intellectuals can be suddenly disturbed by emotional outbursts. The untrained intellect has no power to check emotion. Those who have examined the external world ultimately find that there is something more to know and discover. They then turn within and start understanding their internal states. To do this they first need to make their minds one-pointed, and then become aware of the fact that the emotional level is deeper than the level of thoughts. However, when the mind is made one-pointed and inward, it becomes lost and finds itself incapable of fathoming the deeper and more subtle levels of inner life without the help of emotional power. So one cannot understand his entire personality by means of the thinking process alone, but he can do this by knowing the power of his emotions.

Though emotion is a great power, it needs to be directed willfully; otherwise it disturbs the mind. Our emotional body is like a fish in the lake of life. If the lake is in turmoil, it is impossible for the fish to remain calm and quiet. Similarly, if the mind is in constant turmoil, the emotions can never rest, and one can never use them correctly. The mind and emotions are very close, yet they are different in their functions. In the Sanskrit language the mind is called *manas* and emotion is called *bhava*. Let us discuss the origin of the emotions and see how we can make the best use of this power.

It is *kama*, the prime desire, that creates turmoil in the lake of life. *Kama* is the mother of all emotions. Since desire itself is mixed with selfishness, *kama* does not motivate one to serve others but controls one's life and makes one self-centered. It builds a boundary around one and isolates him from the whole. The more one has that desire, *kama*, the more he contracts his personality and is prevented from expanding his level of consciousness.

So desire is the prime factor of all motivations, and actions are performed according to the types of one's desires. When one wants to fulfill a desire, he thinks, comes to a conclusion, and then acts accordingly. There are a variety of desires—active, passive, positive, negative—in the conscious and unconscious mind and they come up to the surface and disturb the thinking process. But as it is important to understand the thinking process, it is even more important to understand the emotions which can disturb the thinking process. One can easily understand his inner being by finding out what types of desires he has.

All desires arise from four primitive fountains. These are self-preservation, sleep, food, and sex. As far as these fountains are concerned, human beings and animals are alike. A human being sleeps, takes food, has sex, and is always concerned with self-preservation. So also is the case with animals. The difference is that in the animal kingdom, all activities are controlled and governed by nature, while human beings have the willpower to regulate and ultimately control these four appetites and thus they are superior to all living creatures in the world.

The strongest of the four primitive fountains is self-preservation. People are always trying to protect themselves; they are afraid because they don't want to die. In a calamity like an earthquake, I have even seen mothers leave very young children and run away to protect themselves because of their strong desire to live. The biggest fear is the fear of death; it is one thing that haunts us all the time. "What will happen to me if I die, if my wife dies?" Most are insecure all the time because of this fear, but dying is a natural process and all relationships are temporary because of it. This is true; and if the truth makes one insecure, then he is never safe anywhere he goes. Nothing can make one secure if the truth cannot, but the truth is that there is no security anywhere. It is better for one to live with the truth than to live with insecurity, for insecurity that comes from the truth is good, and he will eventually enjoy it.

While all great people have achieved a state of fear-lessness, most people live under the pressure of fear all the time. All fears are self-created; they come from a desire to obtain something which one is not fully equipped to attain. Fears develop in the mind, and if they are not examined and understood, they grow. If one keeps all his fears within, then he will become neurotic. The main root of all dangers is fear and the habit of being afraid actually invites danger. I once had an experience which illustrates this point:

I used to sit on the bank of the Ganges before dawn every day. When the sun rose, I would stand and then sit down again. One morning when I sat back down, someone shouted, "Don't move! There is a snake beneath you!" The moment I heard that, I jumped and ran. Then the snake started chasing me! It chased me for fifty yards.

Later, I went to one of the swamis and said, "This place is very dangerous. There are snakes that chase you."

But he replied, "No. Your mind was chasing the snake, and you were actually mentally dragging it behind you. Your mind was negatively concentrated instead of positively concentrated."

Whenever one has a fear, he is inviting danger by imagining it in his mind and then preparing for it. By doing this, one's mind becomes negatively one-pointed and then that fear is not under his control. When one studies the mind he will come to know the positive and negative aspects it contains. The negative mind has exactly as much power in being destructive as the positive mind has in being useful. That is why fears which are unexamined grow stronger and stronger every day until finally one loses his self-reliance.

One can learn to be fearless, but to develop fearlessness, internal strength is needed because truth and fearlessness walk hand in hand. In order for one to achieve the state of fearlessness, he must first examine the nature and cause of his fears. To examine his own fears closely, he will have to go beyond his thinking process. When he does this, he will find that the greatest fear is that of fear itself. But fear really doesn't exist at all! It is like the darkness which is actually only the absence of light. The sun has never seen darkness. It is he who does not see who is in the dark. So one should learn to look at his fears and examine them properly.

Just as fear can cause discoordination between the mind, body, and senses, similar effects can be noticed from irregularities in sleep, the second primitive fountain. Sleep is a daily feature for everyone from rich to poor, and everyone continues to sleep throughout his whole life. But people do not know why they sleep, and few of them even analyze what it is. Sleep is a great pacifier, a state of rest which restores us every day. It is very important. If one's sleep is disturbed, he will get angry, his nervous system will remain very tense, and he will not work well. If one does not sleep properly, he will be full of fears and will think that everyone is his enemy. If one doesn't get the rest which sleep provides, he will remain in this same mood every day and may even become insane. He will not be able to maintain his equilibrium.

It is very unhealthy to go to sleep when one is upset or has been talking crossly, because such sleep will not be refreshing. One should walk, read, or in some way resolve his differences and try to find solutions for his problems before he goes to sleep. He should meditate or pray, but should not go to sleep with many problems on his mind. The mind should be free from conflicting thoughts before one goes to bed. Going to bed with many unresolved thoughts prompts one to have bad, nerve-shattering dreams. Restless sleep and dreams full of bad experiences are not healthy.

Of all the joys in the world, the most enjoyable is sleep. Two people make love and think that this is their finest joy, but then what do they do? They go to sleep. Sleep is the advanced state of joy, but people do not know how to sleep. In ordinary sleep any harsh sounds will make a bump in the sleep pattern and disturb the sleeper. However, there is one very good technique for sleeping which will avoid this. It is called yogic sleep. This is sleep with full determination, and no matter how many drums are beaten near a person who is in yoga sleep, he won't awaken. No one can wake him except himself.

It is a myth that one should sleep for eight hours a day. The average person who works hard can curtail his sleep to three or four hours, and that will be sufficient. But those hours should be spent in deep sleep, not in dreaming, thinking or waking. Sleeping for eight or ten hours is a bad habit. It wastes much time, and there is so much work to do, the finest being meditation. When one has to plan for the next day, when he has to attain the state of tranquility, why should he waste time in disturbed sleep?

One of the finest principles of good health which is very difficult for modern man is waking up early in the morning. Pick up any book of poetry today; there is not a single poem on the rising sun. It's as if not a single poet has awakened in time to write about the rising sun within the last fifty years. After Shakespeare, Shelly, and Keats, who talks about the morning sun? Recent poets never talk about the dawn. Instead they talk about how beautiful the evening clouds are—sunset, evening dances, evening music—everything is evening and nothing is morning. But one should learn to get up early in the morning. Before the sun rises, one should rise from his bed.

There are certain times in the early morning when the ultra-violet rays of the sun have properties which help the skin. There are skin diseases which cannot be cured by medicine but which can be cured by the sun's rays. So it is very important to wake up in the morning and do exercises before the sun. When one forms the habit of sleeping too long, he is filled with drowsiness, and that habit is called laziness or sloth. By making oneself lazy in this way, he creates much unhappiness for himself.

Food is the third primitive fountain of emotion and poor food habits can make one emotionally upset and physically ill. The first control a teacher will give his student is control of the palate; one should look for the food value

in what he eats, not the taste. In his instructions, the teacher
uses a bitter pill with a blessed effect, but the world uses a
sweet pill with a poisonous effect. One's food habits can
make him emotionally upset, insecure, and sick, but if one
takes food properly, he can avoid this. Being obsessed with
food can have many causes. Sometimes those who do not
eat the food which is essential for their bodies become
emotionally disturbed and think of food all the time. One
may also be compensating for a problem with one of the
other primitive urges by overeating. Some people become
"foodaholics"—they eat constantly. But this is a danger,
because one cannot digest the food properly if the digestive
system is never given a chance to rest. In taking food, one
should examine his capacity, act according to what is helpful
in attaining his purpose of life, and maintain a state of cheerfulness.

Just as one's food should be regulated, so should sex,
the fourth primitive urge. It should neither be overdone nor
suppressed since doing so can create many nervous and
mental diseases. Sex is the least strong of the primitive
urges; it is the only one we can live without. There is no
doubt that sex is a very powerful urge, but it is not the most
important. The reason it often appears to be so important
is because it is more related to the mind than the other three
urges. It is also related to our relationships with other
people. The sex act needs emotional control. People should
prepare themselves mentally and unconsciously for having
sex. A regular date and time should be set for this. By
regulating one's sex habits, one's mind does not run to the

grooves of sexual thoughts all the time.

Sexual obsession and frustration are equally harmful. If one represses himself sexually, or if his sexual life is not happy, this frustration will show itself in actions relating to one of the other primitive fountains, such as overeating. One should analyze his desires and regulate his habits according to his capacity and the purpose of life.

If these four primitive fountains are controlled, they can be the source of good health and longevity and eventually one will be able to regulate his thinking process and all of his emotions. If they are not regulated, they will be the source of many problems and diseases.

One should learn to be peaceful while going to sleep, to be cheerful while taking food, and to be fully under control while doing sex. Otherwise, problems can be created in one's mind. Anyone who wants to enjoy life can enjoy it in a better way if these appetites are regulated. If one has emotional problems, he is making a mistake somewhere in controlling one of the urges, because all problems come from them. It is not difficult to know the source of problems if we learn to observe these four primitive fountains. Those who have regulated the four primitive urges have control over their emotions, and those who have emotional maturity are successful in the world and can be successful in enlightening themselves and attaining the purpose of life, which is self-perfection.

One should learn to observe his capacity and to be aware of one concept: no extremes. Those who are extremists do not know how to establish control over their appetites for food, sleep, and sex.   If one knows how to regulate these appetites, he will surely lead a healthy life. Regulation helps the system and tunes it into the natural laws.   Regulation does not mean abstention; it means balance based on examination of one's capacity. Oversleeping or undersleeping, overindulging in sex or sexual repression, overeating or too much fasting are injurious to one's health. They can damage one's system and his whole purpose in life. They weaken the mind, create guilt feelings and make one lose confidence. When one studies the emotions, he finds that there are seven main streams of negative emotions which arise from the four primitive fountains or appetites. Desire or *kama*, which we have already discussed, is the first stream and the mother of them all.

Anger is the second stream of negative emotion flowing from the four primitive urges. It is the expression of frustration for a desire which finds obstruction in its fulfillment. One should try to remember this whenever he gets angry and to understand that anger is different from what many modern therapists suggest.   They say, "Come on, release your anger. Let it out."   It is true that if one is not allowed to express his anger, it will turn into another disastrous direction; so one can let it out momentarily for the sake of his health. However, when one becomes angry, his nervous system is activated and in the fit of anger a human being may start acting like a wild animal. If one were to get angry all the time, he would want to express his anger all the time and there would be no end to it. He would be forming a very bad habit. Anger is such a blind emotion that at its peak, one can commit suicide or kill others. If one were allowed to release all his angers, he would be behind bars in a day. All the negative emotions are blind, but anger is the most dangerous.

Therefore, it is very important to know how to train oneself not to get angry. This can definitely be done and it will happen when one learns how to control his desires. One should decide which desires are helpful for his growth and which desires will create obstructions to his growth. Learning to train the intellect within (*buddhi*) will definitely help in doing this. If one has not developed this ability and he gets angry, by sitting down and analyzing why he got angry in the first place and examining which desires were not fulfilled, he can arrive at the source of his frustration and anger.

The third stream of negative emotion which is harmful for unfoldment arises when one's desire is fulfilled and he becomes proud. "I have fulfilled my desires and others could not fulfill theirs. Look at how great I am." Pride happens when one has something others do not have and he is constantly aware of this.

The fourth emotion occurs when someone else succeeds in attaining the object of one's desire and he does not. This is called jealousy. One may have something, but someone else may have something he thinks is better. He finds himself incapable of fulfilling his own desires if the other person is fulfilling his. When one is jealous, he is condemning himself for being incompetent. He has lost the battle and accepted defeat.

The fifth emotion comes when one has something and he becomes attached to it by identifying himself with it. He doesn't see its true nature—that it will go to decay, to destruction, to death. He becomes so attached that he doesn't realize this. For instance, a man has a wife and as long as she is fulfilling all his desires, he remains pleased with her. But the moment she loses her beauty, he gets upset. This is called attachment. Nowadays people do not seem to know the distinction between attachment and love. Attachment is selfish; love is selfless. Attachment brings bondage; love gives freedom. Attachment contracts consciousness; love expands it. Attachment becomes a source of torment; love becomes a source of liberation.

When two people meet, they should come together in grand liberation and joy, not in bondage and attachment. Misery comes because of attachment, because there is no giving in the relationship. The greatest happiness in life comes from giving, and the greatest chaos comes when two people claim to love each other but are really attached. Such a relationship which is built on expectation can only bring misery. When one really learns to love somebody, he will be doing things selflessly and spontaneously, for love is that concern in which one enjoys giving and doesn't expect anything in return. That is the way to freedom.

The sixth emotion comes from attachment. It inspires one to want more and more. It is a perverted cultural desire which comes through competition and insecurity. It makes one narrow, selfish, self-centered, and petty-minded. It is called greed. Greedy people do not want to share the object of their attachment with others; they want to protect it.

The seventh emotion is the last and most powerful. It is the egotism which leads one to separate himself from the whole by comparing himself to others. Many times this is based on false pride. One is afraid because there may be somebody better than he is. People who don't have anything frequently become egotistical to compensate for their inferiority complexes.

By examining these seven streams of emotion—desire, anger, pride, attachment, greed, jealousy, and egotism—one can analyze himself. By studying one's thoughts, speech, and actions, he can find out how emotionally mature he is. All control is emotional. If the emotions are not controlled, there is no control at all. Control does not mean suppression of expression; it means regulation and balance within one's capacity. With the help of reason and observation one can remain beyond the sway of emotion.

One should learn to attain a state of emotional maturity in which he knows how to use his emotions positively. Positive emotion leads one to self-reliance and self-confidence, and motivates mind, action, and speech in a joyous and creative way. Unselfish love is the highest positive emotion, and it can lead to devotion. When one loves another, he wants to serve and give to the loved one. He is prepared to give that person anything he possesses. Such joy is a positive emotion and helps one in being creative and in becoming a success in life. It results in peace, tranquility, and equilibrium. Positive emotion is very helpful in self-growth. It has its roots in selfless service and love for others.

This expands the human consciousness. When the mind tires of analyzing and searching for the answer to certain problems, positive emotion can help and lead the mind to a state of attainment. Those who are "insiders" and know the value of life with its currents and cross-currents, understand that the inner world has much to offer, and the more they dive deep into the inner levels, the more they become aware of their human resources. When the four primitive urges are regulated and the seven streams of emotion are controlled, the positive emotions emerge. Then an aspirant can make best use of that power which is the highest of all human powers and he can attain the highest of wisdom. One should learn to attain a state of emotional maturity in which he knows how to use his emotions positively.

By training oneself on the level of desire, one can come to understand his inner nature. When he does this, he will become aware of that which is called conscience and when one understands his conscience, he will realize that it is like a mirror which can never lie. If one tells his conscience, "I am a liar, but you must say that I am not a liar," his conscience will not be able to do it. If one paints his face, his mirror will always tell him which color it is painted. Even if the whole world tells someone what a wonderful person he is, his conscience will know if he is a fake, and no matter how much one implores it to lie, his conscience will still tell him the truth.

Modern man is trying to kill his conscience. He relies on the feedback from others and is afraid of becoming aware of himself as he really is. This is because as one learns to understand himself from within, he first comes in touch with that part of his personality which he has been condemning, and then he identifies himself with these negative thoughts. Such negative thinking is a constant source of disease. Condemning oneself and continually saying, "I'm sorry," creates a sorry personality and a sorry state of health. Every time one feels bad and sorry, he should learn to recognize and appreciate his own inner potential. One's internal and external conflicts weaken him until he has no capacity to enjoy the qualities within himself.

One should never condemn himself for thinking a particular thought. If one thinks of killing somebody, he should remember that he is not actually killing anyone; he is only entertaining a thought, and he can let it pass away. One should not identify himself with his thoughts. No one is a criminal for having bad thoughts. He becomes a criminal when he identifies himself with those thoughts and starts acting according to them—but not before that. If one lets the thoughts pass away, they are gone. So the thing for which one condemns himself is really nothing. There is no way to overcome self-condemnation except to rely on one's own inner mirror which is called conscience. Going against one's conscience is suicide.

Not a single emotion exists that is not related to something else. There is always some external object involved. Not a single emotion is one's own. When one takes in a sensation, the sensation finally leads to emotion. Emotion means relationship, and relationship means life. As long as we do not participate in life, we will all remain lonely. Loneliness is the root cause of many, many diseases. In a way, everyone is lonely. Though they are admiring and hugging each other, claiming how much they love and are loved, people are actually lonely. If one analyzed that loneliness he would find an amazing thing. He would find that it is those who love him who make him lonely. No stranger has the power to do that. One's loneliness means that his emotions are not under his control, that there is something wrong in his relationships. One should learn to be strong. Strength means not to be influenced by the suggestions and influence of others, especially by their negative suggestions. Positive suggestions become part of learning, but negative suggestions become part of self-destruction.

One can analyze any emotional problem he has, but analysis alone is not going to transform his personality if he doesn't train himself. Following his conscience will help him to appreciate himself and keep him from doing further damage, and that is also a good beginning, but it will not undo the habits that are already formed. So one needs to have a self-training program to change himself. If he doesn't, he may know his problems but he will not be able to get rid of them. For instance, if one knows that his pain lies at a specific spot, that knowledge is not going to help him much. He must learn the way to eliminate it. Everyone already has that ability within, and needs only to become aware of the inner reality and come in touch with those potentials which will lead to a state of perennial happiness.

7
Self-Training

All human beings want to attain a state of happiness which is free from all pains and fears. This can be attained by practicing a self-training method. The ancients described such a program in the traditional yogic manuscripts, and it provides one with a way to reach a state of health on all levels. In following this program, one learns through direct experience, and that alone is valid; it cannot be challenged by anyone. Most people are influenced by the opinions of others, and they hardly take the opportunity to form their own opinions. Suggestion has been the very basis of modern life, and few of us draw our conclusions from direct experience. But without having direct experience, the information that we gather from external forces always remains questionable. That is why modern man needs confirmation. Even in our relationships at home we expect others to tell us that it is good to do this or that. "You look good. Your clothes are nice. You speak well." These expressions show that modern man constantly seeks the confirmation and appreciation of others because he is not sure on his own that he does well. Once someone has direct experience, however, he will be sure of his own actions.

Direct experience does not need any evidence to prove its validity. When one has direct experience, no external force can ever influence him, no matter how strong it is. The suggestions and opinions of others will not affect one then, for knowing alone is not true knowledge. One obtains true knowledge only when he starts experiencing. So in the program described by the ancients, one is actually his own textbook, and he compares his own experience with that of the sages to verify the theories they give.

Self-training for self-knowledge works through experience, and although it is very subtle, it can bring one to the finest level of understanding possible. It is the best of all therapies. As human beings, we all need it because we do not know what situations may arise in the future, and we should be fully equipped to cope with them, whatever they may be. In a self-training program, one trains himself. He is his own master and his own student. He plays both roles. If the student is very conscientious and the teacher is very honest, then they can grow together.

For many years, I have worked with people in therapy programs. They all start out by saying, "Okay, let me see the doctor." But no health program in the world will ever be successful if the patient remains dependent upon the doctor, because then the patient will always be a patient and the doctor will always remain in the role of doctor. If one wants to train himself, books, teachers, and other external aids are fine, but one has to learn for himself. He has to involve himself in a learning program. Getting training from a teacher, going to a seminar for a few days and then saying, "It was good; I learned many things," is not completely helpful in itself, even if it was an inspiring program. One is still not fully educated. The real program for self-education begins when one starts adding to these external sources himself, getting into it, feeling, participating, realizing.   Otherwise, happiness, perfection, and *samadhi* are just words which are read in books. We know how to spell them, but we do not grasp their meaning. A human being has all the resources within needed to attain the highest state of wisdom.

If one does not study himself through direct experience, he will be dependent all the time on the opinions of others. He will never have a chance to experience the cause of things for himself. For example, someone goes to his teacher and says, "I had a psychic experience; what do you think about it?" The moment he asks the question or seeks confirmation, it means that there is some doubt in his mind, but an experience which is conclusive in itself does not need any verification. It becomes the guide of one's life. Then one can become fearless. One should go through self-examination, self-analysis, and self-training, for this is the simplest way to gain self-understanding and perfect health on all levels.

One of the greatest problems in human life is that we are often motivated to do things without fully understanding why we are doing them. People are always suggesting that we do things. For instance, if one is in pain, and there is no doctor around, everybody will tell him about some medicine he should take or some special treatment he should have.

He becomes caught up by their suggestions and doesn't use his common sense. He doesn't use his own mind to decide for himself what he should do. One should not allow himself to become dependent upon the opinions of others. He should do what he thinks, not what others think. Yet neither should one be so egotistical that he fails to hear and evaluate suggestions, since proper interaction with others is also very important.

One should accept the idea that he will train himself, but he should not make any big resolutions. Small things are the best to start with. To begin with, one should improve himself by learning to be kind and gentle right at home with the people he loves. A husband should be a very good husband, and a wife should be a very good wife. Just trying to do that is a sign of growth. One should let those he loves see these signs of growth, and then watch his own development and enjoy it. Just as one watches a child grow, one should learn to see his improvement growing as a little spiritual child inside himself. Practicing spirituality should not cripple one's daily duties. He should practice assimilation, gently adopting new habits to help his spiritual growth.

If, for the sake of practice, one divides his life into two worlds, internal and external, then progress will become very easy. He will find himself in a situation of gradual transformation, not of sudden change. One should not expect change; he should not expect that after working with himself his appearance will change. That will not happen. But transformation is possible. Transformation is not change; it is growth. When one learns to transform his personality, then he will understand both his inner conditions and the world around him.

The first day one practices, he will discover that his personality is made up of the thinking process, or outer life, and the emotions, or inner life. One should leave the inner personality aside at first and deal with the external behavior. In this way, he can direct his mind, action, and speech. One should learn to speak less and not jabber uselessly. When one directs that energy which is now running along many avenues to the external world, he can do what he wants. Sometimes merely a wish will make something happen, for that wish can be so powerful that the event will take place of itself. Nothing happens in the external world that has not already happened in the inner world. A plant will not sprout if the seed has not already begun to grow inside its shell. All things that are happening on the outside have happened within long before. But willing something and using willpower are two different things. For instance, if one wills to do something, and then cannot do it, it is because there is no power supporting that will. There is no determination. If one has firm determination, with no distraction and no obstruction, then his willpower can create anything in the world.

When I was young, I once asked my master, "What is free will?" He said, "Go and stand there." So I went and stood firmly on my two legs. Then he said, "Stand on one leg." So I did it. Then he said, "Now lift both legs."

I said, "It is not possible!"

He said, "You have fifty per cent of your will at your

direct disposal. So first you should learn to use that. The other fifty per cent will come to you when you have learned to use the first fifty per cent." When one wants to do something and cannot find the power to support the will, then it doesn't happen. When there is power behind it, then it happens. So learning to use one's free will with determination and creativity is the next step in training oneself.

Whenever a problem comes up, one should not try to escape from it. He should learn to face it. When he faces it, he will find that it is not so bad, but if he tries to escape from it, it will create more and more problems for him. Wherever one goes, he will find new disturbances, but he cannot anticipate what those problems will be. One cannot escape from the disturbances of life, so running away will not help. Therefore one's problems should be faced boldly and honestly.

Next, one should learn to be honest with himself. This does not mean that one should be selfish. Being honest means learning to listen to oneself from within. In fact, the purpose of all the great scriptures of the world is to help one be aware of and in touch with that part within which is called the conscience. Their purpose is to introduce one to himself, to that part of himself which only he can know. Following one's conscience strengthens his power of intuition. It is the first step towards spirituality.

After this, one should learn the philosophy of love or detachment. This will bring peace. This does not mean renunciation or depriving oneself of the things of the world, but it does mean not being absorbed by the world, not being

lost in it. One should remain above. Then he can love anything that comes to him as a means to gain his goal. No
matter what happens, one should be constantly aware of his
goal to maintain tranquility. One should learn to balance the
world within and the world outside, but he must understand
more about his inner world because he is a citizen of that
true inner origin. If one relates to people properly, does his
duties in the external world, knows the art of living in
the external world, and is still not happy within, then he is
not balanced, for he is not tranquil and cannot be considered
to be a whole person. Tranquility does not come from either
isolating oneself from or losing oneself in the world. These
two extremes are not healthy for human growth. One's
attitude in the external world should be balanced, and in the
internal world one's awareness of the center of reality should
be increased more and more and more. It is easy to act in
the external world if one can remain aware of the reality
within. So he should learn how to perform his actions while
remaining aware of this inner reality all the time.

There are two principles which can help one do this.
The first is to become self-reliant. If one is not happy, he
should not expect others to give him happiness. Happiness
can never be given by anyone. This is the only concept
which can help one be happy in the world and if one doesn't
grasp it, if he doesn't really learn it, then he will never be
happy. If anybody claims that he can give someone else
happiness, it is not true. Nobody can give happiness to
anyone. They can only create patches of happiness for
them. It is just as if something should happen to one's

own house. A neighbor might come and help him patch it.
But if one depended too much on others, after some time he
would be thanking everybody and those thanks would
become a curse. He would realize that his whole house was
nothing but patches and that it was no longer a sound structure. One day it would collapse. So one should do the
rebuilding himself and not depend on others; otherwise
he will let himself become a house of patches. He should
be self-reliant and learn how to make himself happy. Many
people expect others to make them happy, but they are
never happy no matter how much others try to please them.
Life is not limited to only the span that is seen. It is a long
procession from the unknown to the unknown. Happiness
is an attitude of mind coming out of an internal state of
tranquility that allows one to go through that procession
without disturbance. But if one is expecting pleasure, he is
also bound to have pain. Life is like a coin of which one
side is pain and the other pleasure. One should realize these
two inseparable opposites and accept life as it is. If one
learns to be self-reliant, then he will be happy.

Practicing an internal dialogue is the second principle
which can help one remain aware of the reality within
while he is doing his actions in the world. One should sit
down every morning and talk to himself. This will help him
learn more about himself, and knowing about himself, he will
not become egotistical. All the ancient scriptures are dialogues. Christ talked with His apostles; Moses talked with the
wise men; Krishna talked with Arjuna—these are all dialogues.
We should also learn to go through a mental dialogue of our

own. One could ask himself, "Am I right? Am I really being fair?"

"Why do you feel bad? People say you are bad, but do you think you are? Do you want to accept this?"

"I think I have been bad, but it hurts me. I don't want to admit it."

"You are afraid of being hurt, and you don't want to realize that fact. This means you are weak."

"So how can I have strength?"

"Perhaps you should be honest. This dishonesty is draining your strength."

You should have this kind of dialogue with yourself within your mind every day. A conscious process of inner dialogue like this can pacify one and wash off all his bad feelings. This dialogue is one of the finest therapies there is and prepares one for meditational therapy. Meditational therapy, if used and understood properly, is the highest of all the therapies and teaches one how to be still on all levels: how to have physical stillness, a calm and even breath, and a calm, conscious mind. Then by allowing the unconscious mind to come forward, one can go beyond it, and that inner reality comes to the conscious field and expands. One cannot explore the totality of the mind unless he applies the special technique called meditation, and unless he uses that inward method, he will never be able to understand himself within. He will not be able to communicate, to relate to the external world, or to use his intelligence in a creative way. This ability comes through involving oneself in a self-training program.

When one begins to explore that inner world, he realizes that the world within is larger than the world outside. One's outside world is actually very small, but when he closes his eyes, he can travel in his inner world to the sun, the moon, the stars. One can travel anywhere mentally and he doesn't need anyone's help. He can create a great world within himself, and it can have many levels. First of all, one comes in touch with the world of his own thoughts, but from where do those thoughts arise? It is like standing by the side of a lake and throwing a pebble into the water. That pebble will create many ripples, and after it has gone down to the bottom of the lake, it will create bubbles. These bubbles will come up again and make more ripples. In the external world a sensation is just like a pebble in the lake of the mind. It leaves an impression within our minds and creates many bubbles; when it leaves a permanent impression, we call it memory. When one is pursuing meditational therapy, he first comes in touch with those memories which are fresh. Then he comes in touch with those memories which are old, and then he comes in touch with those formless memories which are sleeping within, which he has not been aware of until this time. Facts without forms cannot be remembered unless one comes in touch with that part of the mind which is called the hidden mind, and when one comes in touch with that, it leads the way. When one experiences this, it is like the fog rolling back from the world and into the ocean. An unborn chicken which remains inside the shell can never imagine what is outside, but when the shell is broken, the whole situation changes. One should learn to break that shell that he has created around himself, for creating boundaries contracts the personality.

How does one realize that fact, that reality which is beyond names and forms? When one's mind is prepared for it, then he will start treading the path of spirituality and start enlightening himself. This comes through one's direct experience from within. It is not a creation; it is not an attainment. How do we know what enlightenment is? We know because the great people who were born just like us, whose mothers were just like our mother, who walked on the earth, who were human beings, but who had enlightenment, told us what it is and how to reach it. Human beings do not understand that they are complete. They doubt their own existence but they want to believe in the existence of something which they have not realized, felt, or seen. They should learn to believe, appreciate, and admire their own existence first. That is what proves the reality of the existence of the Lord.

We are each a part of eternity. If God is omnipresent, then He is within us too. The day we come to know that all these boundaries are created by self-ignorance, absent-mindedness, and selfishness is the day we can break them and just be enlightened.

My master used to say, "You are already God, so don't try to know God. That godly part is already there in you. All you have to do is become fully human. That is your part to play—to be a good human being so that the reality called God can flow spontaneously." Human beings act abnormally and try to get enlightenment without understanding what it is. The greatest misery is that each of us has a home but has forgotten the way to get there. One does not identify himself with the reality of God within. He only identifies himself with that which seems to be convenient, which seems to comfort momentarily. But after going through many experiences in life, one comes to know that though he has a body, he is something far beyond it.

Enlightenment is an expansion of consciousness. When one becomes enlightened he becomes aware of something more than himself, of something more than his own interest. The more he becomes aware of others, the closer he comes to the center where he finds that all diversities have an underlying unity. The diversities are only superficial layers of the one unity. There are many ornaments, but there is only one great goal. There are many waves, but there is only one water. All human beings are different, but they all inhale and exhale the same life force. No matter what religion one comes from, there is only one proprietor of all the different beings. When one considers this reality for some time, one starts thinking, starts understanding, starts becoming aware of the truth. If one wants God to reveal himself, he will, but first one has to create the proper conditions. If you were to go to the powerhouse with a light-bulb in your hand and ask, "Will you please light my bulb?" they could not do it. The power outlet is in your own house. This is where you have the switch and all the fittings. So why do you need power from outside when it is already there inside you? The powerhouse is within you. It is ready to give you power, but only when you have all the proper fittings. You are shouting, "Oh powerhouse, oh, powerhouse, please come to me!" But it is already there! All you need are a few of the fittings.

When you have truly understood yourself, you are one with the source of peace, bliss, and perennial happiness within. You have reached that state which is called enlightenment, and when you have done this, you become an instrument which can be played by the source within. When you play the guitar, you have to tune it first and that is a painful thing for the guitar. If you really want to be enlightened, be prepared for this. All the parts of your body will have to be properly twisted and tuned because He wants to play. You cannot be selfish. If you are selfish and resist, you will break. You are exactly like a guitar which is being played. If you just let yourself become a willing instrument, there will be no problem.

Sri Swami Rama

Swami Rama was born in 1925 into a learned Brahmin family in the Indian state of Uttar Pradesh. Orphaned in childhood, he was brought up in the cave monasteries of the Himalaya Mountains by a revered yogic sage of Bengal, and was ordained a monk in his early teens. As a young man he was involved in an extended learning journey, studying and living with more than one hundred sages in the solitude of the Himalayas as well as on the plains of India.

From 1939 to 1944 he taught the Upanishads and Buddhist scriptures in various schools and monasteries while studying philosophy and psychology at the universities in Varanasi and Prayag. He earned a medical degree from Darbhanga Homeopathic Medical School in 1945, and then studied Tibetan scriptures in Tibet from 1946 to 1947. In 1949 Swami Rama became the Shankaracharya of Karvirpitham. This is the highest spiritual post in India, but in 1952 he renounced this high office and dedicated his life to creating a bridge between the East and the West by establishing a center of learning from where the message of the Himalayan sages could be faithfully delivered.

He has founded numerous centers of the Himalayan International Institute of Yoga Science and Philosophy in

India, Japan, Europe, and the United States. Dedicated to the benefit and edification of all humanity, the Institute offers a wide variety of educational, research, and therapeutic programs. Swami Rama is the author of many books, including *Living with the Himalayan Masters, Lectures on Yoga, Book of Wisdom, Freedom from the Bondage of Karma, Life Here and Hereafter,* and *Inspired Thoughts of Swami Rama.*

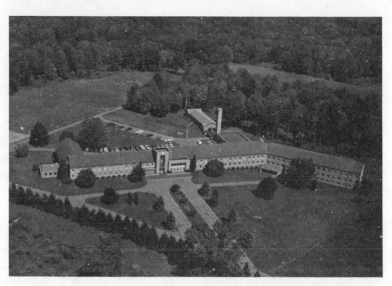

The main building of the national headquarters, Honesdale, Pa.

The Himalayan Institute

The Himalayan International Institute of Yoga Science and Philosophy of the U.S.A. is a nonprofit organization devoted to the scientific and spiritual progress of modern humanity. Founded in 1971 by Sri Swami Rama, the Institute combines Western and Eastern teachings and techniques to develop educational, therapeutic, and research programs for serving people in today's world. The goals of the Institute are to teach meditational techniques for the growth of individuals and their society, to make known the harmonious view of world religions and philosophies, and to undertake scientific research for the benefit of humankind.

This challenging task is met by people of all ages, all walks of life, and all faiths who attend and participate in the Institute courses and seminars. These programs, which are given on a continuing basis, are designed in order that one may discover for oneself how to live more creatively. In the words of Swami Rama, "By being aware of one's own potential and abilities, one can become a perfect citizen, help the nation, and serve humanity."

The Institute has branch centers and affiliates throughout the United States. The 422-acre campus of the national headquarters, located in the Pocono Mountains of northeastern Pennsylvania, serves as the coordination center for all the Institute activities, which include a wide variety of innovative programs in education, research, and therapy, combining Eastern and Western approaches to self-awareness and self-directed change.

SEMINARS, LECTURES, WORKSHOPS, and CLASSES are available throughout the year, providing intensive training and experience in such topics as Superconscious Meditation, hatha yoga, philosophy, psychology, and various aspects of personal growth and holistic health. The *Himalayan News*, a free bimonthly publication, announces the current programs.

The RESIDENTIAL and SELF-TRANSFORMATION PROGRAMS provide training in the basic yoga disciplines— diet, ethical behavior, hatha yoga, and meditation. Students are also given guidance in a philosophy of living in a community environment.

The PROGRAM IN EASTERN STUDIES AND COM-PARATIVE PSYCHOLOGY is the first curriculum offered by an educational institution that provides a systematic synthesis of Western empirical sciences with Eastern introspective sciences using both practical and traditional approaches to education. The University of Scranton, by an agreement of affiliation with the Himalayan Institute, is prepared to grant credits for coursework in this program, and upon successful completion of the program awards a Master of Science degree.

The five-day STRESS MANAGEMENT/PHYSICAL FIT-NESS PROGRAM offers practical and individualized training that can be used to control the stress response. This includes biofeedback, relaxation skills, exercise, diet, breathing techniques, and meditation.

A yearly INTERNATIONAL CONGRESS, sponsored by

the Institute, is devoted to the scientific and spiritual progress of modern humanity. Through lectures, workshops, seminars, and practical demonstrations, it provides a forum for professionals and lay people to share their knowledge and research.

The ELEANOR N. DANA RESEARCH LABORATORY is the psychophysiological laboratory of the Institute, specializing in research on breathing, meditation, holistic therapies, and stress and relaxed states. The laboratory is fully equipped for exercise stress testing and psychophysiological measurements, including brain waves, patterns of respiration, heart rate changes, and muscle tension. The staff investigates Eastern teachings through studies based on Western experimental techniques.

Himalayan Institute Publications

Living with the Himalayan Masters	Swami Rama
Lectures on Yoga	Swami Rama
A Practical Guide to Holistic Health	Swami Rama
Choosing a Path	Swami Rama
Inspired Thoughts of Swami Rama	Swami Rama
Freedom from the Bondage of Karma	Swami Rama
Book of Wisdom (Ishopanishad)	Swami Rama
Enlightenment Without God	Swami Rama
Life Here and Hereafter	Swami Rama
Marriage, Parenthood, and Enlightenment	Swami Rama
Emotion to Enlightenment	Swami Rama, Swami Ajaya
Science of Breath	Swami Rama, Rudolph Ballentine, M.D., Alan Hymes, M.D.
Yoga and Psychotherapy	Swami Rama, Rudolph Ballentine, M.D., Swami Ajaya
Superconscious Meditation	Usharbudh Arya, D.Litt.
Mantra and Meditation	Usharbudh Arya, D.Litt.
Philosophy of Hatha Yoga	Usharbudh Arya, D.Litt.
Meditation and the Art of Dying	Usharbudh Arya, D.Litt.
God	Usharbudh Arya, D.Litt.
Yoga Psychology	Swami Ajaya, Ph.D.
Foundations of Eastern and Western Psychology	Swami Ajaya (ed.)